Health writer Paula Goodyer is a Walkley
Award-winning journalist and former
health editor of *Cleo* magazine. She is the
author of *BodyGuard* and *Kids & Drugs*.
She has two daughters and lives in Sydney
with her partner, photographer
Rick Stevens.

An Ebury Press book
Published by Random House Australia Pty Ltd
Level 3, 100 Pacific Highway, North Sydney NSW 2060
www.randomhouse.com.au

First published by Ebury Press in 2009

Addresses for companies within the Random House Group can be found at
www.randomhouse.com.au/offices

National Library of Australia
Cataloguing-in-Publication Entry

Goodyer, Paula.
Fit & firm forever.

ISBN 978 1 74166 583 3 (pbk.)

Physical fitness for middle-aged women.
Strength training for women.
Menopause.

613.7045

Cover concept by Christabella Designs
Cover photography by Kiren Photography Productions
Internal design saso content & design pty ltd
Typeset in Minion 12/17pt by 1000monkeys.com.au
Printed and bound by Griffin Press, South Australia

Random House Australia uses papers that are natural, renewable and recyclable products
and made from wood grown in sustainable forests. The logging and manufacturing processes
are expected to conform to the environmental regulations of the country of origin.

10 9 8 7 6 5 4 3 2 1

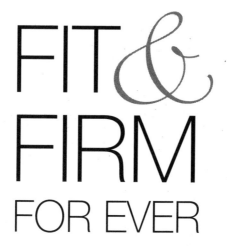

FIT&
FIRM
FOR EVER

Paula Goodyer

EBURY
PRESS

To my mother, Joan Goodyer,
and my grandmother Annie Platts –
two strong women who never sat around.

Contents

PART TWO DIET AND LIFESTYLE

Introduction

Midlife expansion: who stole my waist?

I'm at a party one Saturday night when suddenly it dawns on me that almost every fiftyish woman is wearing a jacket over her dress. It's not because it's a particularly chilly night but because, as men in suits have always known, jackets camouflage a potbelly without making you look like a dag.

Forty might be the new 30, and 50 the new 40, but one thing doesn't change: menopause still arrives at the usual time. We might have redefined middle age and look a decade younger than our grandparents did at midlife, but the same biological clock ticks on, ringing in premenopausal changes from the mid-40s onwards. With it can come the feeling that your shape is out of control. Why, when you could win back your waist after a pregnancy or two, can the run-up to menopause make it harder to stay slim?

For most women, menopause happens somewhere between 45 and 55, and this ten-year period is also the prime time for female weight gain. Over this decade women typically stack on around five kilos: around half a kilo a year. Much of this extra fat ends up around the waist and it's not a good look – hence those jackets.

But it doesn't have to be the downhill run to easy-fit pants and big girls' blouses. Although about 50 per cent of Australian women over 45 are now overweight or obese, there's no law of nature that says this is inevitable. For most of us, there are no mysterious biological forces beyond our control that mean we'll never look decent in a good pair of jeans or a pencil skirt again. Middle-age spread is an option you don't have to take.

But first things first. To win back your shape – or keep the one you've got – it helps to know what can cause the female body to change its shape in our 40s and 50s.

There's no mystery about why extra weight at middle age hangs around the waist – it's all to do with hormonal changes at midlife.

When a woman's body is in its younger, baby-making phase, the hormone oestrogen encourages extra fat to be stored around the hips, thighs and butt – it's nature's plan to ensure reserves of fuel to help women survive and care for her kids if the food runs short. (In fact, as you'll read later, it's nature's little tricks for ensuring survival of the species that have a lot to do with many of our weight problems.)

But by the mid- to late-40s, when levels of oestrogen start to drop, any surplus fat can start settling around the waist instead. It's the start of a process which, if you let it continue, gradually erodes your shape.

With fat settling around your middle – but less padding on your hips, butt and thighs – the curve between waistline and hips starts to vanish. That's when you suddenly realise what a great asset hips are – they accentuate your waist and give your body shape. There are more insults to your contours ahead – if muscle loss increases, your butt will get flatter as you get older, leaving a space in your jeans where the curve used to be.

But although there's a biological reason for *where* the fat ends up, it's not absolutely clear why this extra weight creeps on in the first place – although many researchers believe an activity deficiency, not a hormone deficiency, is a likely cause.

There's currently a large study of around 40,000 Australian women underway that is gradually building a snapshot of women's health at different ages. It's called the Women's Health Australia Survey. When the researchers looked at the data relating to menopausal women, they found that not all of them gained weight. The difference between those who gained weight and those who didn't was that the non-gainers reported doing more vigorous exercise – they also avoided the kind of food traps that contribute to kilo creep, such as eating high-fat snack foods and takeaway foods. Over in the US it's a similar story. Research has found that women going through menopause, who are physically active, have smaller waists and gain less weight than those who aren't active.

What's also interesting about the women in the Australian study is this: while the weight gainers were more likely to put their extra weight down to factors beyond their control, the non-gainers were more likely to be taking steps to keep the kilos off.

But aside from the vanity issue, a bulging mid-section at 45+ is also a risk factor for a bunch of health problems you want to avoid – think high blood pressure, heart disease, stroke, diabetes, sleep apnoea, fatty liver disease and cancer.

While we're used to hearing about the connection between being overweight and heart disease or diabetes, not everyone's aware that, next to not smoking, sticking to a healthy weight is one of the most important ways of preventing cancer. Being overweight is now linked to a number of cancers, including the women-only kind like post-menopausal breast cancer and endometrial cancer (cancer of the lining of the womb). Nine per cent of breast cancers diagnosed after menopause are thought to be caused by obesity. Why carrying extra fat boosts breast-cancer risk after menopause isn't known, but a prime suspect is fat's role in producing oestrogen – too much of this hormone may promote the growth of cancerous cells in the breast.

But the good news is that losing your shape isn't inevitable – knowing that midlife is prime time for weight gain gives you a head start – you can take action now to hold on to your shape.

Women's bodies do come in all shapes and sizes and it's crazy to compare ourselves with images of celebrity bodies that have often been surgically sculpted or airbrushed to perfection.

That being said, loving your body also involves loving it enough to care about its health and wellbeing. If you've been lucky enough to be born with a healthy body, then along with that comes a responsibility to keep it that way – and this book will show you how.

If this is your problem ... here's your solution.

A **thickening waist and/or belly bulge** You can avoid midlife belly blowout by eating better and becoming more active – especially if you're prepared to add some strength training to regular 'cardio' exercise like walking, running, cycling or cardio classes at the gym. Besides being a fabulous all-round body toner, strength training helps you lose weight more effectively, and – as you'll learn in *Fit & Firm* – brings a heap of extra health benefits too.

Flabby, flappy upper arms If you're generally overweight, then shedding some kilos will help trim the flab in this trouble spot, while simple strength-training exercises will tone up the triceps muscle at the back of your upper arm. (You'll never need to hide under long sleeves again.)

Droopy boobs You can perk up the muscles in your chest, creating a lifted, more youthful look, with anti-gravity exercises that target your upper body. The combination of toned upper arms, chest and shoulders is a winner in tank tops and strappy dresses – and subtracts years from your age.

Shapeless butt You've heard about middle-age spread, but did anyone warn you about MSBS – Menopausal Shapeless Butt

Syndrome? The combination of muscle loss and the hormone changes that encourage weight to settle around your waist rather than your lower body can flatten your butt. Learning to do squats and lunges with weights can make a difference by pumping up the butt muscles.

Pudgy thighs Firm them up with walking, jogging or cycling, combined with muscle-toning exercise to firm up your thighs. Besides better looking thighs, you'll have legs that work better – the benefit of stronger legs is that they help you walk further without getting tired, keeping the rest of you fitter and firmer too.

Bra fat All-over weight loss, together with strength training, will make a difference to those fatty overhangs that creep up on you in your 40s and 50s – though it's hard to wipe out bra fat entirely. Even if you're skinny, the lessening elasticity of your skin can still create some spillage over the side of your bra, but wearing stretchier bras that don't dig into your flesh should help minimise the overhang.

Drooping posture Strength-training that targets postural muscles in your back and shoulders will help keep you erect. Good posture really matters at 45+ because it helps combat the overall droopiness of a woman's body, which starts to kick in at menopause as muscle loss increases.

Part One

Fitness

Chapter 1

Are you ready to re-style your body?

Remember when 'looking good for your age' meant the Joan Collins school of age defiance – taking how you looked at 35 and freezing it by painting over the lines with make-up, and/or resorting to a nip and tuck? We've all seen on TV that this can look pretty peculiar, as ageing beauties begin to resemble weird caricatures of themselves at younger ages.

But if we had to pick just one powerful thing out of all the therapies, products and techniques touted as anti-agers, which works better than anything else, it would be regular exercise. You can tinker around the edges of your body with firming cream, seaweed wraps and spa treatments – but what makes a major difference to how your body looks and functions is never something you do lying down in a salon or a spa for a few hours. It's what you do – usually on your feet – walking, cycling, jogging, swimming, dancing, stretching or strength-training *on most days of your life.*

Sure, there's always those seductive ads for cosmetic surgery and the promise of losing love handles via liposuction without burning a single kilojoule – but what can lipo or a scalpel do to boost your defences against heart disease, diabetes and dwindling bone strength? Nothing. The right kind of exercise, on the other hand, has the power to lift, trim, tone, strengthen, reboot your energy – *and* prevent chronic illness, all at the same time.

Sydney personal trainer Sheryl Macrow-Cain says that women who start taking their fitness seriously in their 30s are often the ones who reach peri-menopause (the run-up to menopause) in their late 40s feeling more in control of their bodies.

'I think being overweight ages you – it's so easy to look frumpy because you can only wear certain clothes,' says 55-year-old Sydney business educator Anne Riches, who whittled her wardrobe of size 14s and 16s down to size 8s and 10s through a combination of Weight Watchers and distance swimming. She swam the two-kilometre Cole Classic ocean race near Sydney's Manly Beach by training with Can Too, a Sydney-based organisation offering free professional training in running and swimming endurance events to people of all ages. In return, participants raise funds for cancer research by joining in community running and swimming events.

It was looking in the mirror and feeling fed up that motivated Anne to lose weight. 'Clothes shopping had become a problem – they don't make fashionable clothes for 50-something women in size 14s,' says Anne, who's always liked swimming but had never tackled long distances. After only a month of training, she could swim two kilometres. She now works out six times a week – five swims and one session of strength-training and stretches.

'They're strong, they're in good shape and they have terrific bone density,' she says. 'Yet it's not a message that's getting out to younger women – at 35 they think they can get away with being inactive, but they're not looking further down the track.'

It's not rocket science that being physically active helps fend off weight gain by burning up kilojoules. But there's another way that exercise, especially more vigorous exercise, can make a big difference – it helps stop your basal metabolic rate from slowing down, a problem that many researchers now believe is a fundamental cause of weight gain at menopause.

The basal metabolic rate (BMR) is the rate at which your body burns up kilojoules when you're at rest, as opposed to moving around. Not long ago, a slow BMR was considered an inevitable part of getting older – but not any more. Now it's thought to have more to do with the gradual loss of muscle brought on by declining levels of activity as we get older.

10 compelling reasons to exercise

Your body looks so much better in clothes (and without them)

There's no shortage of good advice on how to look good naked in women's mags and on the net – get a spray tan, get a body scrub, get waxed, get moisturised, get a pedicure. Nothing wrong with that, except there's something missing on this list – a regular appointment with exercise. It's working out over the long haul that helps keep weight off permanently – not just for a few weeks or months.

It helps boost your sex drive

Even if no-one had bothered to study the link between exercise and sexuality, it would make sense that something that keeps your body working better, your energy levels higher and your stress levels down can only be kind to your sex life. But another reason why research suggests exercise enhances sexuality is because it makes people feel good about themselves and increases their confidence. A study of female students in the US found that most of the women who rated their fitness level as high, rated their sexual desirability as above average – or much above average. This resonates with something a 48-year-old triathlete once told me. 'Exercise just makes your whole body hum with energy,' she said. 'And that flows into everything else you do – including sex.'

Exercise can help reduce menopause symptoms (without any scary side effects)

Some research suggests that women who exercise more have fewer hot flushes – no-one really knows why, but one theory is that it's because exercise reduces stress, which is considered a trigger for hot flushes. A recent Spanish study looked at two groups of women aged 55 and older. One group did no exercise, while the other spent 12 months on a program of cardio work, strength-training and stretching. At the end of the 12 months the number of women with severe menopausal symptoms in the group of exercisers had gone down – but among the non-exercisers, the numbers had gone up. Interestingly, the women who gained weight in the Women's Health Australia Survey mentioned earlier also reported more hot flushes and night sweats. This doesn't mean that staying at a healthy weight is an iron clad guarantee of a cooler menopause, but it comes with so many other health benefits that it's definitely worth a shot.

It may delay biological ageing

Forget cosmetic surgery – go for a jog instead. Keeping fit with aerobic exercise (walking, jogging, cycling, cardio gym classes) through middle age and older can hold back biological ageing by about 12 years. Fitness tends to fall steadily from middle age so that it gets harder to do everyday activities without getting tired – but according to a *British Journal of Sport Medicine* report, regular aerobic exercise slows this process down. It may be that being physically active somehow delays the ageing of our cells too. If you haven't heard of the term 'telomere' yet, you will soon. Telomeres – stretches of DNA on the end of our chromosomes – are attracting scientific interest because of their link to ageing and cancer. Telomeres have been compared to the protective plastic tips at the end of shoelaces that prevent the laces from fraying. Each time one of our cells divides, the telomeres get shorter. And when they get too short, the cell can't divide any more and dies – a process that's been linked to ageing and cancer. Now here's the good news: UK researchers have found that people who are physically active have longer telomeres than couch potatoes.

It buys you time

A 30-minute walk or a workout at the gym might seem like one more thing that's impossible to squeeze into your day – but do it often enough and you'll become more productive. Physically, you get more done when you're fitter and stronger, while the oxygen boost to your brain helps you think better too. Walking and running can also de-clutter your mind, giving you good thinking time to problem solve, make plans, or just give your brain a break.

It makes you healthier – even if you're overweight

What if you needed to lose weight and improve your health, but could only choose one way to do it – more exercise or a healthier diet, but not both? Exercise would be the best pick. No one's suggesting you don't do both, but it underscores how incredibly valuable exercise is. An overweight person who exercises can have a lower health risk than someone of normal weight who does no exercise.

Even if you're overweight and you find that walking for 30 minutes a day makes little or no difference to your weight, you're still getting a benefit because it's reducing your risk of heart disease and other problems. A sedentary woman with a size 8 wardrobe who eats very little might think she doesn't need exercise – after all, she's not overweight. But exercise isn't just about dress size – she still needs exercise for her health's sake.

It's like an all-purpose health pill

It's impossible to ignore the mounting evidence that exercise prevents or helps to treat a long list of diseases. The proof of its power is now engraved in Medicare – people with chronic health problems including high cholesterol, insulin resistance, diabetes, depression and osteoarthritis are now eligible for a Medicare rebate for consultations with an exercise physiologist who can plan an exercise program for them. Regular exercise can also boost your immune system so you're less vulnerable to colds and flu.

Your heart will last longer

The list of heart benefits of an exercise habit is long – regular exercise lowers the risk of clots forming in the arteries. It also encourages blood vessels to make nitric oxide that helps keep arteries supple. Researchers looking at the link between exercise and the risk of heart disease and stroke in women aged over 45 in the US Women's Health Study found that women who exercised the most were 40 per cent less likely to have a heart attack or stroke than those who did the least amount of exercise.

Exercise helps keep blood sugar levels healthy too. The more active you are, the more your muscles soak up glucose to use for fuel, and that's good news for arteries – high levels of blood sugar encourage bad LDL cholesterol to form plaque in artery walls.

It brings the pressure down

Exercise reduces blood pressure by making your heart stronger. And the stronger your heart is, the less effort it takes to pump blood around your body. This means there's less pressure on your arteries.

Your brain will get fitter

Intuitively, it makes sense that what's good for your heart is also good for your head – clean, unclogged arteries that keep blood flowing to your heart will also keep your brain cells supplied with the nutrients and oxygen it needs to stay in good shape. This may partly explain why more and more research suggests that regular exercise seems to reduce the risk of dementia (especially if it's vigorous and includes strength-training) and improve memory. With the help of imaging technology, scientists can now look into living brains to get a better idea of the effect exercise has on it. When researchers from the Columbia University Medical Center peered at the brains of a group of people who'd been working out for three months, they discovered they'd grown new nerve cells. The brains that grew the most new cells belonged to the people who'd become the fittest. Other research suggests exercise can enlarge the part of your brain responsible for 'executive function', meaning important mental tasks like planning, decision making and multi-tasking. This is also a region of the brain that's thought to deteriorate with age.

What kind of exercise is best?

The one you like the most and is the easiest to fit into your life but, for the best results in terms of good health, healthy weight and a better, more efficient body, it's best to try and combine the following three different types of exercise:

* *Aerobic* (cardio) exercise to burn kilojoules and make you fitter
* *Strength-training* to increase the number of kilojoules you burn, and to shape your body
* *Flexibility exercises* to keep your body supple.

Ten minutes to a better butt, and other myths

Just as all children must learn there is no Santa Claus, all smart women must learn that magazine cover lines can lie. Despite what the glossies say, you can't drop a dress size by Friday, or get the body you want in ten minutes a day. You could get a better butt in ten minutes a day though – *if* that means ten minutes of lunges and squats as part of a regular 45-minute workout two or three times a week, with some walking or running thrown in.

So how much time do you need to spend on exercise? That partly depends on what shape you're in to begin with, how sedentary you are, and how much weight you need to lose. On average, it's best to aim for an hour a day, six or seven days a week. There's a great research project in the US called the National Weight Control Registry that tracks the habits of thousands of successful 'losers' so that the rest of us can learn from what they do. The participants are people – and mostly women with an average age of 45 – who've kept weight off for at least five years, and 90 per cent of them exercise for an average of an hour a day.

Thirty minutes exercise a day has been the loudest message from Australia's official physical activity guidelines since the late 1990s. It's a great place to start if you're not active at all, and helps lower your risk of heart disease and diabetes. But, if you have a sedentary job or you need to lose weight, it doesn't go far enough. If you check out the full guidelines, you see that the 30 minutes they specify is the *bare minimum* we should do daily, not the grand total, and that the guidelines include other pieces of advice that don't get heard as often, including:

- 'If you can, also *enjoy* some regular vigorous activity for extra health and fitness' This is another way of saying it's a smart idea to do something more intense than walking a couple of times a week, like going for a run, jumping on a bike, playing tennis, or doing a class at the gym.
- 'Be *active* every day in as many ways as you can' In other words, your daily activity quota shouldn't stop at 30 minutes a day.

Thirty minutes a day can only do so much. It was designed to coax couch potatoes out of their chairs, improve their health and help reduce their risk of heart disease and diabetes – all of which it can do. But it's not going to shift much weight or help maintain a healthy amount of muscle, especially as you head into your 40s. If you ask the man who wrote those physical activity guidelines back in 1999, Dr Garry Egger, Adjunct Professor of Health Sciences at Southern Cross University, he'd be the first to tell you that 30 minutes is no longer enough.

'If I were asked to rewrite the guidelines now I'd double the 30 minutes a day to 60 minutes, and recommend some kind of resistance (strength) training every other day,' he told me in an interview for *The Sydney Morning Herald*.

What has happened in the last few years to make him change his mind? There are two things. First, there's the recent scientific research that shows a stronger link between physical activity and health (the fact that strength training can help prevent diabetes is one example). The other major factor is the ever-increasing use of the internet. 'Having the world at our fingertips' means we've lost even more reasons to move.

Make exercise a habit you can't give up

The right exercise can work miracles for health and looks. But to make it work it has to be as routine as brushing your teeth – something that most of us do because the alternative to not cleaning them is so much worse: sick gums and teeth that look bad or fall out of our heads. We need to apply the same routine maintenance approach to exercising our bodies, given that the alternative to not exercising is pretty similar – bodies that look bad, get sick and don't last as long.

Whether it's eating healthily or being more active, half the battle is organisation and time management. In the following chapters you'll find options for getting fitter, stronger and leaner. But before you jump in and make choices, think about how you'll fit an exercise routine into your life – and how you'll maintain it.

If you're over 40 ... See your doctor for a check-up before you start exercising, especially if you have any risk factors for heart disease. The factors include being overweight, smoking, high blood pressure, high cholesterol or diabetes. (Even if you weren't planning to get fitter, this age is the prime time to get these checks done.) And don't forget the Medicare rebate that's available for people with some chronic health problems. You can see an exercise physiologist and get advice on how to be active. See the Australian Association for Exercise and Sports Science website at www.aaess.com.au.

Fitting exercise into a busy life

What really pays off in terms of a healthier, better looking body is putting in time and effort. That doesn't mean you wake up tomorrow and run a marathon – it means you start off slow and easy and gradually pick up the pace as your fitness, strength and energy levels increase.

But reaching this goal will cost you around six hours a week of planned exercise and you have to figure where those hours will come from. You don't want to short-change yourself on sleep (often a recipe for low energy and overeating, as you'll read later in this book), so where else can the time come from? You could:

- *Watch* less TV (it's no coincidence that successful weight losers on the National Weight Control Registry mentioned earlier watch less than ten hours of TV a week).
- *Exercise* in your lunch hour.
- *Get up* earlier (but go to bed earlier too).
- *Slot in* 20 to 30 minutes exercise by walking part of the way to work.
- *Delegate* more. If you're a woman who shoulders much of the burden of cooking and cleaning up around the house, it's time to off-load some of it on to the rest of the family. Getting others in the family to fix dinner a couple of times a week can free you up to go for a walk, a run or squeeze in a cardio or yoga class. And if you feel a stab of guilt, remember that people who are in good shape physically and mentally do a better job of looking after others.
- *Bring* exercise and family together. If it's hard to do more exercise without compromising time with family, get them to join in!
- *Find* ways to bring more movement into your free time. There's no rule that says your social life must be conducted sitting down around a table – meet people for coffee and a walk. Join friends at weekends to do something active – like a Sunday morning walk followed by breakfast together, or a bike ride or a swim.

Even walking around a museum, an art gallery or window-shopping is good – not as intense as a 30-minute brisk walk or a run, but it beats sitting.

* *Use* the weekend to make up for lost time if there's less time to exercise in the week – longer walks or runs, or double-up with a walk and a strength-training session on Saturday or Sunday. Or be more adventurous and have a stab at different kinds of activities that you can do with family and friends too – like hiring kayaks or trying indoor climbing.

When's the best time for more exercise?

The morning?

There are good reasons for exercising first thing in the morning – it's over and done with before anything crops up to interrupt your plans. If you want to burn fat, morning workouts have some advantage over an evening session – after a 30-minute run your metabolism can be elevated for up to eight hours, helping you burn more kilojoules during the day, points out James Short, a Sydney-based personal trainer and past President of the Fitness NSW Personal Trainers' Council. That said, the best time of day is the one that's easiest for you to fit in – and different times have different benefits.

Lunchtime?

Rather than make you feel tired, exercise – once you're used to it – can recharge you, so if you can squeeze exercise into your lunch hour, you'll work better in the afternoon. Is there a gym close to work? Can you walk for 30 minutes at lunchtime – or even organise a lunch hour walking group at work? You need to fit in time to eat too, so bringing in lunch from home will save you time. Remember that if you run rather than walk in your lunch hour, you'll need to eat afterwards, not immediately before – but it's best to have a carbohydrate snack (a piece of fruit is enough) about an hour before you go.

Late afternoon / evening?

The advantages of exercising later in the day are that your muscles are warmer, it helps you relax and put the working day behind you, and gives you an energy boost for the evening ahead. (Just don't exercise too late in the evening – working out too close to bedtime can make you too wired to sleep.) It's ideal if you can head off for a walk, run or a gym class straight after work – it makes a good dividing line between work life and home life. But if demands on your time at home are almost as heavy as those at work, you'll need to do some forward planning, or delegate dinner to another family member. Failing that, you can always walk for 30 minutes after dinner and do some strength training, followed by some stretches while you watch TV.

Tips for keeping an exercise habit

- *Make* exercise a priority – not an afterthought.
- *Schedule* exercise time in your diary.
- *Try* to have at least two weekly sessions firmly embedded into your routine so they're unlikely to be disrupted. Scan your weekly schedule for time slots on two or three days when plans are least likely to be derailed. Let family and friends know these are your regular walking/running/gym times so they understand that you're not available. This way these sessions will become a habit.
- *Have* a back-up plan for when exercise plans get derailed. For example, if your plan to walk at lunchtime has to change, what can you do later in the day instead?

'What would I say to a 40-something woman who said she couldn't run? I'd say, "You have no balls, you have no imagination – don't limit yourself",' says Gina, a 50-something ex-smoker. 'I was 51 and knew I had to give up smoking so I decided to run the City to Surf – but, at that time, I couldn't even run to the corner of my street. I set myself small goals – by the end of the following week I'd be running for five minutes and by the end of the month, I'd be running for 15 minutes. I also set myself a reward – I'd buy myself some Bulgari earrings if I could keep going for 20 minutes. But then I decided to push myself a bit more, I'd have to run for 30 minutes before I got the earrings.'

By the time she could run for 20 minutes, Gina hired a personal trainer who helped increase her fitness with the help of interval training – alternating short bursts of faster running with her usual jogging pace.

'Sometimes I thought I'd die, but I decided I'd rather die running than die of smoking. It really helped me quit because I realised how much smoking could affect my lung capacity. Without running, I don't know that I would have given up smoking.

'Most women of my age are putting on weight, but I can eat what I want and drink champagne,' says Gina, who now runs for 45 minutes three or four days a week, often as part of a group training session.

'I like the social contact of a group, and people who run together give each other a lot of support and encouragement to keep going.'

Why you can do more at 45+

To shed weight and improve the way your body looks, you need to begin with your head. Some people have a habit of psyching themselves out of physical activity as they move further into their 40s. It's as if they mentally shrug themselves into an old cardigan and decide there are things they can no longer do. It's not helped by the fact that golf and gardening have become synonymous with suitable activities for the over

50s. These, of course, are perfectly okay things to do, but it's sending the message that crossing the line from the 40s to the 50s means you're incapable of anything tougher than a gentle stroll. The reality is that women in their late 40s, 50s and older are out there lifting barbells, paddling kayaks and running (ask anyone who's competed in a fun run and I bet they remember being overtaken by someone in their 50s or older). As you face another birthday, it's not necessarily your age that decides what you can and can't do.

Exercise physiologists – health professionals who are experts in human movement – now think in terms of a person's functional age. This means taking into account how active they are and what they can do physically – rather than assessing them on their chronological age. Chris Tzar, Director of the Lifestyle Clinic at the Faculty of Medicine at the University of NSW says there are few physical activities that our 'birthday' age stops us from doing. It's more about identifying any health problems and getting expert advice to help you exercise safely.

How you use your body at the age you are now will influence how well you live the next few decades of your life. But even if you're a sloth now, you can still turn an inactive life around – research has shown that even people who don't become physically active until after they've turned 40 are 55 per cent less likely to develop heart disease than people who stay inactive. And while the standard advice for becoming more active is to choose walking, preferably with two strength-training sessions each week, don't assume you can't do something more strenuous, just make sure you take it slowly.

We do not stop playing because we grow old; we grow old because we stop playing.

Benjamin Franklin

Action list

- Accept that not exercising is simply not an option at 45+.

- Don't accept that a pudgy waistline is part and parcel of menopause.

- Look at your weekly routine and decide where to slot in exercise time. You may have to create time by cutting back on TV time or cooking time (there's nothing wrong with salad and a can of tuna).

- Overdue for a check on your blood pressure, cholesterol and blood sugar levels? Get it done – it's important to know what the numbers are (and if they're too high, that's more motivation to be more active).

Chapter 2

The miracle of muscle

Creeping muscle loss begins in your 40s and, with each passing decade, you'll say goodbye to about three kilos of muscle, which is then replaced by fat – unless you do something about it. Vanishing muscle has more to do with weight gain than you think. The amount of muscle you have affects how well your body burns energy – the more muscle you have, the more efficiently you burn kilojoules. The reason for this is that fat and muscle behave differently – muscle burns up more kilojoules than fat – so the more muscle you have, the more kilojoules you can chew up, even when you're just sitting. But when you start losing muscle and gaining fat, you burn fewer kilojoules and gain more weight.

There is also another way that dwindling muscle can make it easier to add extra padding around your waist. Less muscle means less strength, and less strength means any physical activity feels harder and tires you out faster. This sets up a vicious circle: the harder the physical stuff gets, the less you want to do – and the less active you are, the weaker your muscles get.

This isn't a signal to take things easy and do less – it's your body begging for help. It needs you to do more to boost its muscle strength so it can move around more comfortably. Moving less will only speed up muscle loss and make it harder for your body to burn kilojoules.

US research following more than 3000 women aged 42 to 52 bears this out – while it found that many women gained weight and added centimetres around the waist at this age, this was related to how much, or how little, they were exercising.

'It was the strength-training that really stripped the fat away,' said Lee-Anne Carson, aged 50. 'Women think it's normal to have flab under their upper arms as they get older, but it's not. I don't have tuckshop arms any more. When I look in the mirror I see toned muscles,' says Carson, a business development manager living in Sydney. Her moment of truth came after overhearing her teenage son describing his mother to a friend: 'She's blonde, wears glasses and she's fat.'

Ten kilos overweight, with climbing levels of both blood pressure and blood sugar and a family history of heart disease, Lee-Anne had seen her weight gain accelerate in her 40s, especially around the waist.

'I was starting to look old,' she says. 'I was looking into the mirror and seeing my mother.' Eighteen months later, she's swapped her size 16s for a size 10, and both her blood pressure and blood sugar levels have dropped down to normal levels.

Four months after turning up (terrified, she admits) for her first training session with Can Too, she finished a half-marathon. She's now completed three half-marathons and a one-kilometre ocean swim.

'The running has been great, but I think it's the strength training that really strips the fat off and makes you really toned,' she says. 'I don't jiggle any more – and my husband says I've got runner's legs.'

Still, showing up at the gym to do weight training wasn't easy for her at first. 'I contacted a personal trainer – but I cancelled six appointments before I finally turned up to keep one. I felt fat and I found the gym unnerving, but I kept telling myself, "Who cares that you're fat – you have the same right to be here as anyone else."'

When you dig into the biology of why ageing makes human bodies look old, it's not hard to see why exercise is the nearest thing to a youth drug.

The reason a 60-year-old body looks different to that of a 30-year-old isn't just the wrinkling of its outer skin, it's what's happening to the stuffing inside – when muscle and bone start shrinking and muscle gets replaced by fat, bodies sag and posture droops.

The good news is there's an antidote: boosting muscle strength. Not long ago, scientists thought that the gradual muscle loss that starts in the 40s was an inescapable effect of ageing that put you on the downhill run to frailty – in a body increasingly made up of more fat and less muscle.

But strength training can reverse muscle and bone loss, making bodies work better, shed weight and stay leaner. In fact, strength-training does such wonders for women's bodies that if it came in a cream created by Lancôme and promoted by Angelina Jolie, we'd splurge half a week's salary on a 250 ml tube.

Besides sculpting your body in a way that aerobic exercise alone can't do, working out with weights (just light ones to begin with) is an investment in long-term health. While it works to make you look good on the outside – trimming muffin tops and jelly arms – it's also working on the inside to help prevent thinning bones, rising blood pressure, high cholesterol and diabetes.

What's miraculous about muscle is that it's one of the few things that affect how we look where you can actually *undo* some of the effects of ageing. When hair goes grey there's no way to put the colour back naturally. Lose teeth and you can't grow them back. But muscle is different – if you're prepared to put in some work, you can replace much of the muscle you've lost over the years so that your body works better and looks better. In other words, it's possible for some aspects of your body to actually improve without the help of scalpels and anaesthetic. With strength training, helped along by a healthier diet and cardio exercise, your body gets firmer, not flabbier, and it functions better. Women who work out with weights two or three times a week can lose around a kilo and a half of fat in two months, according to research – and for each half-kilo of muscle gained, they burn about 140–200 kilojoules more each day. There's even some evidence that strength-training can actually reverse muscle ageing. If you did high school biology you'll recall that your body's cells contain something called mitochondria, which produce energy to keep the body running. It's mitochondria's slow deterioration that's thought to nudge along the ageing process. But Canadian researchers found that in a group of 65-year-olds, six months of twice weekly strength training reversed the deterioration of the mitochondria in their muscles.

Whatever age you are and whatever shape you're in – either perfectly formed or very overweight – you'll benefit from stronger muscles.

Let's just suppose weight is not an issue for you; you can grab a size 8 or 10 off the rack and know you'll slip into it without straining to close the zip. But you still need to build muscle – because under your skin you're gradually losing muscle and, sooner or later, this loss will start to show up. Your body might be slim but it will gradually acquire a droopy look, as more muscle is replaced by fat, and the muscles that help support your posture begin to shrink.

It's also true that as women's bodies age there can come a time when they fall into one of two camps: matronly (because they're carrying extra weight) or scrawny (because they've stayed skinny). Carrying some extra muscle can help you tread the line between the two – lean enough not to look matronly, but with enough 'stuffing' to not look like an old chook.

So, if strength-training can do so much, why are many women scared off by the idea of working out with weights?

Probably because the image of strength-training is still tainted by images of bodies bursting with muscle. If you talk to many women about lifting weights, they think of muscle-bound men or freaky women with oiled bodies and cricket-ball biceps. If you suggest that they build muscle or strength, a lot of women back off, as if picking up a barbell will transform them into Karen the Barbarian.

This is partly because people confuse strength-training with body building. But there's a big difference – body building is more about creating exaggerated muscle definition by inflating muscle size and reducing fat to a bare minimum for competitions. That muscle-bound look involves specialised diets and heavier weight training.

But while women who strength-train might want to look a certain way too, it's a different look – firm and toned, not knotted with muscle. Fitness instructor Sally Hitchman, who's been teaching strength-training at Sydney gyms for 15 years, says that although it's not hard to get women to turn up for strength-training classes with names like Body Pump and Body Blast, it's often hard to persuade them to increase their strength by lifting heavier weights. They usually baulk at the idea. Hitchman says, 'Some women also psych themselves out of working harder because they don't believe they're capable of being strong.'

It's for this reason that some personal trainers and gyms simply play down terms like strength-training or weight training in favour of the less intimidating 'toning'. Yet Hitchman isn't muscle bound – neither are other women I know who strength-train – but what they all have in common is that they're in terrific shape. These women don't go shopping for clothes that hide a bulging waistline and they're flaunting sculpted upper arms at an age when other women's triceps have turned to porridge.

Apart from what muscle can do for the look of your body, it's also smart to be strong at midlife. If you were to guess which physical features would be high on most women's wish lists in their 40s and 50s, you can bet strength wouldn't be up there. All our lives we learn that we should have great hair, good boobs, booty that's not too big but not too small, and decent legs. But strength? No, that's not really our department – men need strength and women need strong men.

This might have made some sense back in the days when marriages were made for ever and there was a good chance there would be a man about the house for most of a woman's life. However, with the rise of singledom and higher divorce rates (plus the fact that women generally outlive men anyway), this makes no sense at all. Being strong is *useful* – and if you think about it, don't women have *more* reason than men to boost their strength? Women have about one third less muscle than men to begin with, so when their muscle strength dwindles with age, they get frailer faster.

I also believe that, after thousands of years of being told they're the weaker sex, many women don't believe they have the physical strength to lift weights. Thankfully, no one's expecting you to bench press a bus – as with anything else, it's better to start off small and progress gradually. If you can lift shopping, you can lift a light dumbbell or barbell. No one starts off hefting huge weights – you start off light and build up your strength.

Midlife muscle – why you need it

Muscle can build curves – not bulk

Women don't produce enough of the male hormone testosterone to grow muscles like a man so, while strength-training can sculpt your body, building muscle tone and definition, it's unlikely to add bulk. Apart from anything else, the muscle that you're adding is often muscle that you're meant to have but that you've gradually lost over the decades. But what you *can* gain is a better shape. Remember how one effect of menopause is that you carry less fat around your hips, thighs and butt? That might seem like good news at first – until you realise the shape of your butt is more flatbread than bun. Check out the rear view of most women over 55 and you'll get the picture – but strength-training exercises that work the butt go a long way to preserving its shape.

Working out with weights gives your upper body a lift

Because breasts themselves have no muscle, no amount of strength-training will pump them up or hike them higher, but your chest *does* have muscles and working out with weights can give your upper body a lifted look that looks good in tank tops and strappy dresses, especially combined with the toned shoulders and firm upper arms that come with regular strength-training. Another bonus: upper-body exercises that also strengthen and tone your back and shoulders can have the effect of making your waist look narrower.

More midlife muscle means less midlife fat

Up until about 15 years ago, aerobic exercise like running, walking and cycling were seen as the top fat burners – and they are really good. But what's more effective still is the combination of regular aerobic (cardio) exercise and strength-training. While running, walking, cycling or a cardio class at the gym help you shed kilojoules (and boost cardiovascular fitness), two or three sessions of strength-training a week will give you the edge by helping you burn more kilojoules.

'Strength-training is very effective for weight loss, especially lifting lighter weights for a higher number of repetitions, because after each session of strength-training, your metabolic rate is increased for up to 16 hours, making you burn more kilojoules,' says Sydney strength coach Tony Boutagy, a lecturer with the Exercise Science Department at the Australian Catholic University.

Doing a mixture of cardio and strength-training in one session can help you fast-track fat burning – if you do some strength-training first, followed by cardio work like running or brisk walking, for instance. What's good about doing strength-training first is that it uses up fuel stored in your muscles called glycogen so that when you move on to doing cardio your body will start burning fat for fuel.

The gym is one place to do this – after your strength session you can jump on an exercise bike or a treadmill for 30 minutes. Or, if you've got the hang of using weights by yourself at home, you can follow a 20-minute session with a run or a brisk walk.

You can produce more of your own anti-ageing hormone – HGH

Touted as an anti-ageing drug and performance enhancer that reduces fat and boosts muscle, Human Growth Hormone (HGH) in its manufactured form is one of the most stolen drugs in the world.

We all have our own supplies of HGH (produced by the pituitary gland in your brain), though after peak production in your mid-20s, it declines gradually, dropping sharply after the age of 50. It's this drop that's thought to contribute to the ageing process.

If you can increase production of HGH naturally with strength-training, then there's less loss of muscle mass, better bone strength and less fat, says Tony Boutagy, explaining that when exercise stimulates a release of HGH, the hormone helps your body build more muscle tissue – and use up more fat.

Any vigorous exercise can stimulate HGH production, but strength-training gives the biggest boost – the 'burn' felt in your muscles when you lift a weight repeatedly is a sign that you're producing HGHs, he says. Studies show that it takes about 50 minutes of fairly intense strength-training twice a week to get that HGH spike. And because it's produced when you exercise vigorously, more HGH may be another perk of interval training – the technique of alternating your regular pace with give-it-all-you've-got bursts of more intense exercise.

Stronger muscles mean better bones

Boosting bone strength isn't just about eating more yoghurt (though that helps). The kind of exercise you do really matters too. The downhill run to thinning bones starts around the mid-30s when bone strength peaks – after that you lose bone mass by about half to one per cent a year up until menopause. After that it's more like one to three per cent a year. Your bones' worst enemy is inactivity because it makes them weak. By tugging on the tendons that anchor muscles to bones, strength-training stimulates bones to grow.

Dr Maria Fiatarone Singh, now Professor of Medicine at the University of Sydney, and Dr Miriam Nelson of Tufts University in the US, compared a group of 50- to 70-year-old women who lifted weights twice a week, with a group of women who did no exercise. By the end of a year, the women who exercised had maintained their bone density, while the non-exercisers had lost about two per cent of theirs.

Muscle helps protect your heart

It's not news that aerobic exercise like walking and running can help prevent health problems – but in the last decade there's been a new recognition that strength-training has big health benefits too – that's why the American Heart Association and the American College of Sports Medicine now say adults need two weekly sessions of strength-training, as well as regular aerobic exercise. Apart from shifting waistline fat, strength-training can improve heart health in other ways. Boosting leg strength makes it easer to walk faster and further, giving heart and lungs a better workout. strength-training can also lower blood pressure, as well as levels of bad LDL cholesterol, which directly benefit the heart.

Extra strength can improve your blood sugar levels

Strength-training can help prevent diabetes because it increases muscles and reduces abdominal fat. To understand the link between muscle and diabetes, it helps to know that your muscles soak up blood sugar to use as fuel. The more muscle you have, the more blood sugar they take up, and the less risk of having high blood sugar levels that can lead to diabetes (remember how strength-training helped normalise Lee-Anne Carson's blood sugar levels earlier in this chapter).

On the other hand, the more muscles shrink, helped along by chemicals produced by fat around your middle, the less blood sugar they use, and the higher your risk of diabetes, explains Maria Fiatarone Singh, an international researcher into the use of strength-training as 'medicine' to treat diabetes, arthritis and osteoporosis.

For people who've already developed diabetes, Australian research by the International Diabetes Institute found that six months of regular strength-training improved blood sugar control by 14 per cent – a result similar to that achieved with medication. If you think this is a non-issue for you because you don't have diabetes, don't be so sure – problems with blood sugar are more common than you'd think and now affect almost one in four Australians over 25 (often without their knowing it). Either they have full blown diabetes or their risk of the disease is higher because their body has trouble controlling their blood sugar levels.

Strong women have more energy

How's this for a sad piece of news? A study of 34- to 58-year-old women by the University of Michigan in the US found that those who lost around 2.5 kilos of lean muscle walked more slowly and had less strength in their leg muscles. That's another way of saying that walking had become harder. These women were hardly ancient, yet muscle loss was already beginning to chip away at their strength. The flipside of this is the more optimistic finding, again from Miriam Nelson at Tufts University. After a year of strength-training, a group of middle-aged women became 27 per cent more active – and leaner too. Gaining muscle makes any physical task easier, whether it's walking, climbing stairs, shopping, lifting, housework, gardening, dancing or playing sport. And who couldn't do with a stronger body that gets more done with less effort?

Yet according to Dr Nelson, 30 per cent of middle-aged women have trouble doing physical tasks like walking a couple of kilometres, carrying a few shopping bags or climbing a few flights of stairs.

Working out with weights gives your mood a lift

Research has shown that strength-training can work just as well as Prozac for improving depression – though for this and other health benefits of strength-training, it should be done at high intensity once you've got the hang of it. The idea is to keep extending yourself so it doesn't feel easy – the equivalent of getting out of breath when you walk.

Exactly how strength-training works to tackle depression is still a mystery, but the educated guess is that it has some positive biological effect on the brain. Unlike cardio exercise, it's not thought to raise endorphins – feel-good brain chemicals – nor is it the social contact with other people, because studies have shown that it works, even when people workout alone.

Strength-training can make you less accident-prone

If you lose muscle strength, you may also wave goodbye to good balance too. There's nothing mysterious about the ageing process that causes so many older women to fall over, often breaking a bone in the process – it's caused by loss of the muscle strength that helps to keep you upright. Strong muscles, on the other hand, help stabilise your body and make it easier to stop yourself falling over if you trip or lose your balance.

Regular workouts with weights can increase a woman's strength by 30 to 50 per cent – something that, in the long run, can reduce the risk of disability and death after a fall.

Boosting your core strength (the muscles in your lower back, pelvis and abdomen) also helps you maintain balance and stability when you move around. Squats, lunges, using a fit ball or doing Pilates are good ways to increase core strength. It's important to activate core muscles by drawing your navel into your spine while doing these exercises.

How good is your balance? Try this quick test.

Stand on one leg with your arms folded over the raised leg, knee tucked toward your chest and see how long you can stay like that without clutching at something for support. If you can do this for 30 seconds you're doing well (even better if you can do it with your eyes closed!) Too hard? Try repeating the test after a few months of strength-training – you should see a difference.

How does strength-training work?

Lifting weights breaks down protein in your muscle fibres – the soreness you feel the next day is caused by tiny tears in the muscles. Over the next few days you lay down more protein in the muscle, and it's this healing process that builds stronger muscles.

As your strength grows, you can gradually increase the amount of weight you lift so your muscles continue to get stronger.

So where do I start?

You can strength train at home by yourself, but it's best to get some expert advice to help you get your technique and posture right. Your options are:

THE GYM

Many gyms run strength-training classes where you lift barbells and dumbbells to music. These classes are easy to follow and it can be fun working out in a group. You don't have to be coordinated or good at sport to lift weights – just copy what the instructor does. They provide a good introduction to strength-training, especially in a small class where it's easy for the instructor to make sure everyone's working correctly. A good instructor will check with people in the class to see who hasn't done the class before and help them use the right techniques (which aren't difficult).

Some gyms offer casual classes – this means you don't need to take out gym membership to join classes. Or you may be able to take out a short-term membership for a month if you don't want to commit to a full-time membership. If you think the gym isn't for you, don't rule it out until you've read page 64. If you're self-conscious about your body or think you'll feel uncomfortable in a unisex gym, look for a women-only gym in your area.

STRENGTH-TRAINING CLASSES AT A LOCAL COMMUNITY CENTRE

Some community centres offer fitness classes including strength-training. Check with your local council to see what's available in your area.

A PERSONAL TRAINER

Personal trainers aren't just for the rich and famous. A few sessions with a good personal trainer can be a great investment in your health and your looks, and help you achieve results you didn't think were possible. While you can get fit without a personal trainer – it's not hard to teach yourself how to run, for instance – with strength-training, it's best to have some expert advice to start you off and help you get the technique right.

If you think paying someone to help you workout is wildly extravagant, think again. It's no more extravagant than paying a hairdresser to give you a great cut and colour, or handing over tuition fees to learn a new skill – which is exactly what strength-training is. And if it's a financial toss-up between having a regular pedicure or manicure and spending an hour with a personal trainer, it's no contest. Nail polish wears off, but with a good trainer you're buying guidance to help you learn to workout effectively so your body will look and function better in the long term.

Fees can vary a lot – expect to pay anything from $50 an hour upwards. It's important to make sure your trainer is qualified and accredited. Suitable qualifications include a Certificate IV in Personal Training or a degree in Exercise Science, and the trainer should be registered with Fitness Australia, the professional body of the fitness industry. You also need to find someone who's right for you, stresses James Short. Things to consider when deciding on a trainer, he says, include:

- ❋ *Will* you feel comfortable exercising in front of them?
- ❋ *Does* the trainer have experience working with women of your age?
- ❋ *Remember* that you don't need a trainer to be your best friend – you want them to motivate you to work and help you reach the level of fitness you want in the safest, most effective way.
- ❋ *Does* the trainer make you feel confident you're in good hands?

To find a registered, accredited personal trainer in your area, contact Fitness Australia, the professional association of the fitness industry, at www.fitness.org.au.

Don't be afraid to talk to a few different personal trainers before you choose the one that suits you best.

GROUP TRAINING

This is a more affordable option than personal training – you workout with a small group of people with one or more instructors, often in public areas like parks and ovals. If you like being with other people, group training could be something you really enjoy.

'The group dynamic helps keep people motivated. You're exercising, but it's social too because you're catching up with friends – it's not like exercising alone on the treadmill,' points out Linda Schlenker, a fitness instructor and director of Step Into Life, which runs group training sessions Australia-wide.

Group training sessions often include a mix of cardio work and strength-training. Costs can vary from $12 to $30 a session. To find group training classes in your area, contact Fitness Australia.

What to expect from strength-training

'In the first two weeks of strength-training, you're likely to feel tired,' says James Short. 'But after this stage you'll start to feel more energetic, and at around six to 12 weeks you'll start to notice changes like less fatigue, and your clothes will feel looser.'

Will it hurt?

It's normal to feel some muscle fatigue when you're working out, or to feel some muscle ache on the first or second day after a workout. But if you're exercising and experience any pain that makes it hard to maintain normal day-to-day activities, then ease off.

You can do strength-training (also called weight training or resistance training) using:

DUMBBELLS AND BARBELLS

These are also called 'free weights'. Their advantage is that they make you use more muscles – including the muscles that help improve posture and balance – because your body has to work to keep to keep the weight stable. You can buy dumbbells and barbells in different weights from a sports store. Dumbbell weights start as light as 0.5kg.

WEIGHTS MACHINES

These are the machines you see at the gym. They can help you train with heavier weights. Because they're so stable, they also allow people with arthritis or little muscle strength to workout in a sitting position until they gain more strength, and they are easier to use.

YOUR OWN BODY WEIGHT

Exercises like push-ups, squats or lunges force you to lift your own body weight, increasing your muscle strength.

The idea is to start off with relatively light weights (nothing you can't handle) and lift and lower them 15 times – each time you lift and lower a weight is called a repetition (or a 'rep'). By gradually increasing the weight of the barbells or dumbbells as you get stronger, you'll build more muscle definition and endurance – endurance meaning that your muscles can do things for longer without getting tired. You'll also find it easier to lose weight or stick to a healthier weight.

A different technique that builds even more strength in both muscles and bones is to lift heavier weights but for fewer repetitions. The idea here is to work up to lifting weights heavy enough so that lifting the last weight is a major effort.

You can also increase muscle strength by lifting the weight of your own body. Try push-ups from the knees or toes to strengthen your upper body or lunges to strengthen and firm butt and thigh muscles.

'Gimme strength' – tips for working out with weights

This section will give you a snapshot of what strength-training involves. Although it could help you workout by yourself at home, its main purpose is to take the mystery out of what's involved and to help you understand the jargon. This means you'll feel more comfortable and be better informed when you start working out at a gym or with an accredited personal trainer – that's how you'll get the best result. If you want to workout with weights at home, obviously you'll need something to lift. You can improvise with cans from the pantry to start with or you can buy dumbbells (hand weights) from a sports store. The dumbbells you use for working out your lower body are generally heavier than the ones you use for your upper body. But it's best to get started by trying a few gym classes. The classes will help you to decide what your best starting weights should be.

WARM UP BEFORE YOU START

This could be five or ten minutes walking, or if you're at the gym you could do five or ten minutes on an exercise bike. If you do a class, the instructor may take you through some basic strength-training moves using light weights as a warm-up.

Whether you're lifting a weight or doing a push-up, the movements should be slow and controlled – this makes the exercise more effective. To give your muscles time to recover and grow, rest one full day between exercising each specific muscle group – e.g. if you do exercises that target the lower body on Tuesday, then do exercises for the upper body on Wednesday. If you work both upper and lower body on Tuesday, skip a day before you workout with weights again.

KEEP YOUR ABS TIGHT AT ALL TIMES

This helps to keep you stable and protect your back.

DON'T 'LOCK' (I.E. FULLY STRAIGHTEN) YOUR KNEES OR ELBOWS WHEN YOU'RE EXERCISING

It can put too much stress on your joints.

REMEMBER TO BREATHE

It sounds obvious – but people sometimes hold their breath when they lift a weight. Breathe out when you lift the weight and breathe in as you return to the starting position.

REMEMBER YOUR POSTURE

Keep your back, head and neck straight.
If you feel pain or discomfort, stop what you're doing.

DON'T ARCH YOUR BACK WHEN YOU LIFT A WEIGHT

If you can't lift without arching your back, use a lighter weight.

START OUT WITH LIGHT WEIGHTS

Not so light that lifting them is totally effortless, but a weight that you can lift 8–12 times.

LOOK AT WHAT YOU'RE DOING IN THE MIRROR
WHEN YOU WORKOUT AT THE GYM

Mirrors aren't there just so people can admire themselves (although that happens); they help you check your 'form'. For instance, if your side is facing the mirror while you do a lunge, you can make sure your torso is straight, and your knee isn't going over your toes.

If you're a beginner, you may find that you're able to lift only light weights, but once your body gets used to the exercise, you may be surprised at how quickly your strength increases. Once you start to find an exercise with a particular weight easy – whether it's an exercise you're doing in a class or one you're doing by yourself – then start using a heavier weight.

Don't be tempted to strengthen just one or two parts of your body – like your thighs, butt or upper arms for instance – otherwise you'll end up with some muscles being weaker than others, and you'll risk injury. Each session should work every part of your body – your chest, shoulders, biceps, triceps, buttocks, thighs, back and abdomen.

REMEMBER TO STRETCH AFTER WORKING OUT

Stretching after a workout will keep you more supple and help prevent post-workout soreness.

- A repetition means doing one single exercise – e.g. a single lunge or a single bicep curl.
- A set means a series of exercises – e.g. if you do a lunge 12 times, you've done a set of 12 lunges.
- Form means technique – if someone has 'good form' when they do a particular exercise, it means they're doing it correctly. Good form is important to avoid injury.

Strong language – how to understand the jargon.

You'll also hear references to different muscles – here are some of the more common ones.

- **Glutes** Gluteal muscles (including the gluteus maximus) – the muscles in your butt.
- **Quads** Quadriceps muscles – the muscles at the front of your thigh.
- **Hamstrings** The muscles at the back of your thigh.
- **Biceps** The muscle at the front of your upper arms.
- **Triceps** The muscle at the back of your upper arms.
- **Abs** Abdominal muscles – these include the rectus abdominus, a large muscle that runs down the abdomen, and the
- **Obliques,** which are muscles that run down the sides of the abdomen.

Basic strength-training moves

There are lots of different exercises that target different muscle groups – this is a snapshot of some basic exercises you're likely to come across when you try a strength-training class at the gym or work with a personal trainer. Knowing what's involved will give you a head start. If you want to try them yourself at home, aim to do each one 15 times (15 'reps' or repetitions). Once you've got the technique right, gradually build up so you can do three sets of 15 repetitions of each exercise. Remember to rest for a minute or so between each set.

Kicking butt

Working the muscles in your butt goes a long way to keeping it firm and curvy. Good activities for this are cycling, lunges and squats. However, if you have problems with your knees, lunges and squats can make them worse, so don't attempt them without talking to an exercise instructor or personal trainer.

LUNGING

Stand with your feet hip-width apart and put one foot behind the other as if you're taking a giant step. Make sure your back foot is quite a long way back. With your back foot, your weight should be on the ball of your foot, with the heel off the floor. Keep your upper body really straight and keep your abs tight (this helps keep you stable). If you need help to balance, hold on to the back of a chair until your balance improves.

Slowly drop your back knee until it's almost touching the floor (or as low as you can go). Stay tall and make sure your front knee doesn't go over your front foot.

With your front heel pushed into the floor, push your body into an upright position. Repeat 15 times on the left leg and then 15 on the right leg. You'll get the most benefit for your butt in this exercise if you squeeze the muscles in your butt as you rise from the lunge into an upright position. That way, you're using your butt muscles to help lift yourself back into an upright position.

You can do lunges with or without weights. If you're not used to lunges it's a good idea to do them without weights to begin with so you get used to doing them the correct way. Even without weights, they're a good exercise if you do them properly but they are definitely more effective if you use either a dumbbell in each hand or a barbell on your shoulders.

SQUATS

This exercise will tone your butt and legs. Stand with your feet shoulder-width apart, knees slightly bent and toes facing forward. Keep your abs tight. Your feet should stay on the floor with your weight pushed into your heels. Lower your butt as if you were sitting on a chair. Lowering yourself so that your thighs are parallel to the floor – but not any lower – will give you the best workout. But be sure that your knees don't go over your toes. Squeeze your buttocks together, using them to push you back into an upright position – the 'squeeze' helps work the muscle in your butt harder.

Like lunges, it's best to do squats without using weights while you get the technique right. When you're ready to use weights you can use a light dumbbell in each hand. Another option (and easy to do at home) is to do squats with an exercise ball placed between the small of your back and a wall. The idea is to keep the ball pressed between your lower back and the wall as you go down into a squat and back up again. You can make this even more effective still if you hold a dumbbell in each hand.

Upper body

Strengthening your upper body helps you sail through everyday activities like lifting, or pushing a lawn mower or a loaded shopping trolley. Stronger, toned shoulders aren't just for men either – they make waists look smaller and balance big hips.

BICEP CURLS

This exercise gives definition to the muscle at the front of your upper arm. Keep your torso and back straight, your elbows close to your sides, your shoulder blades down and your abs tight. With your arms hanging down by your sides, hold a dumbbell in each hand, bend your elbows and lift your forearms upwards so you're lifting the dumbbells to shoulder height. The dumbbells should face your shoulders. Now lower the dumbbell down to the starting position. This should be a slow, controlled movement – don't swing the dumbbell up and down.

REAL WOMEN CAN DO (REAL) PUSH-UPS

I can still remember the buzz of managing my first real push-up – not the kind from the knees, but the real G.I. Jane movement from the toes. It took a week or so of trying – and failing – to lift the weight of my body off the floor with my arms until I achieved it . . . just. By the next day, I could do two. Now, on a good day I can do 20. Or more.

Push-ups might be a symbol of male strength, but they can do great things for the female body – like tightening the flab-prone triceps muscle behind the upper arm, and strengthening and toning the muscles in the chest, shoulders and back. They can also tone your abs – to lift yourself off the floor you need to contract the deep abdominal muscle, the *transversus abdominis* (TA for short), by visualising drawing your navel into your spine.

The great thing about push-ups is that you can do them anywhere, anytime, and you can use different versions to make them harder or easier, and to target different parts of your upper body. *Don't assume that being a woman means you can't do push-ups from the toes* – most women can (they just don't know it). It can take a bit of practise to do your first 'real' push-up, but once you've done one the rest will gradually follow.

Start with modified push-ups, by which I mean push-ups from the knees. This is good for building strength in your arms and upper body so you can eventually graduate to doing push-ups from your toes.

Kneel on the floor, supporting your weight on your hands – keep them slightly further apart than your shoulders. Bend your elbows to the floor and then return to the starting position. Practise until you can do three sets of 8 to 12 with a break in between. For push-ups from the toes, lie face-down with your hands in the same position and your toes pointing downwards. Push your body off the floor and repeat (you'll probably only be able to do one at first – but more will follow). With push-ups from either toes or knees, it's important to keep your abs tight, your head, neck and back in a straight line, and you should aim to get your chest as close to the floor as possible.

TRICEP DIPS

This is an exercise you can do using your own body weight to strengthen and tone the back of the upper arm. Sit on the edge of a step, bench or a stable chair with your hands next to your thighs. Position your hands on either side of your butt on the edge of the bench, fingers facing forward. Lift your butt off the bench and lower it towards the floor by bending your arms at the elbows. Keep your body close to the bench, with your back straight. Lift yourself back up by straightening your arms. Keep your arms close to your body throughout the movement.

SHOULDER PRESS

This exercise helps to tone the upper arms and shoulders. Stand with your feet about hip-width apart with a dumbbell in each hand. Hold the dumbbells up so they're parallel to the floor with one end close to the front of your shoulder. Your palms should face forward. Push the dumbbells upwards until your arms are extended above your head, with your elbows soft (not locked). Slowly lower the dumbbells back to the starting position near your shoulders. When you lift and lower the weight, keep the movements slow and controlled – don't jerk.

UPRIGHT ROW

A great exercise for upper back, shoulders and arms. Standing with your feet shoulder-width apart and knees slightly bent, hold dumbbells side by side at thigh level (your palms facing towards your thighs). Slowly pull them up to your collarbone, until elbows are just above shoulder height. Slowly lower and repeat.

How buff is your back?

It's easy to become focused on what you see when you look in the mirror – but what about your rear view? A strong, toned back looks terrific in summer clothes. Exercises that target the back include anything that makes you squeeze your shoulder blades together. The rowing machine at the gym will help strengthen your upper back and shoulders.

Strong to the core

Your 'core' muscles include the deep abdominal muscles such as the *transversus abdominis* that wraps your body like a girdle, the obliques (the muscles on the side and front of your abs), the *rectus abdominis* – a sheet of muscle along the front of your abdomen (that's the 'six-pack' muscle) and the *erector spinae*, a set of three muscles along your neck to your lower back. Although you can't see them (unless you grow a six-pack), these muscles need to be as strong as any other muscle – they protect your back and improve your balance. Weak core muscles, on the other hand, can be a cause of back pain and falls.

One benefit of strength-training is that many of the exercises, done correctly, also have the effect of strengthening your core. The reason is that you should automatically draw your navel towards your spine ('navel to spine' is a mantra you'll also hear in a Pilates class or gym class) to help stabilise your body. Firmly engaging your ab muscles in this way starts to become a habit if you do it often enough. For your back's sake, it's also important to do the 'navel to spine' move when you lift any kind of weight both in and out of the gym.

Another good way to build core strength is with a fit ball (sometimes called a Swiss ball) but, as with strength-training, it's best to have expert help to learn the basic moves first. Some gyms run fit ball classes and many personal trainers who run outdoor group sessions incorporate fitball training.

THE PLANK

Get on your knees with your weight resting on your knees and forearms, and your elbows under your shoulders. With your toes curled under and heels together, lift your legs, pelvis and torso off the floor, and pull your navel into your spine, while balancing your weight on your toes and elbows. Keep your buttocks in line with your spine and legs and look at the floor. Hold for 30 seconds or longer and repeat three times.

The flat ab kit

You could do a hundred crunches a day and they won't flatten a pot-belly – you'll just end up with really taut muscles obscured by a layer of fat. What works to remove that layer of fat is a combination of cardio work (walking, running or cycling) and strength-training, along with specific exercises – crunches included – that firm and strengthen the abdominal region.

Three things to keep in mind while working on your abs:

Vary your movements

Muscles soon adapt to doing a particular exercise, so it's good to challenge them by changing the way you crunch every few weeks.

Avoid crunching too fast

Crunches should be slow and deliberate. If you do them too fast you're likely to be using momentum rather than muscle to lift yourself off the floor. Try to isolate your abdominal muscles and use them to pull you off the floor, using slow, controlled movements.

Don't lock your hands behind your head to pull yourself up

It hurts your neck and doesn't work your abdominal muscles. Just keep your hands lightly touching your temples.

THE BASIC CRUNCH

Lie on the floor with your knees bent, keeping the small of your back pressed firmly into the floor (this will prevent back injury, especially for novices).

With your hands resting lightly on either side of your head and your elbows back, contract your abdominal muscles as hard as you can and use them (not your shoulders) to raise your shoulders off the floor. Breathe out as you come up – it makes crunching more effective. Pause for a count of one, then lower your shoulders to the floor and repeat. Aim for ten basic crunches, gradually working up to 20.

THE REVERSE CRUNCH

This one tones your lower abs. Lie on the floor with your knees bent in the air, forming a right angle, and your hands at the side of your head. Raise your shoulders slightly off the ground and use your lower abdominal muscles to lift your knees slowly into your chest. Breathe out as you lift, and hold the contraction for a count of one when you've lifted your knees as much as you can. This is only a small movement *using your abdominals only* – no need to lift your pelvis high in the air. Aim for ten crunches, gradually working up to 20.

THE TWIST CRUNCH

This tones the oblique muscles at the side of your waist. Lie flat on your back with your knees bent and your hands by the side of your head. Let your knees flop over to your left side. With both shoulders slightly off the floor, use the muscle on the right-hand side of your waist to lift yourself off the floor. Remember to breathe out as you lift and to hold the contraction for a count of one before you lower your shoulders. Try to do ten, then repeat on the other side. Build up to 20 on each side.

Don't forget your back

The muscles in your back and abdomen work together, so when you've been flexing your abs it's good to balance this with a few easy back exercises. Although these exercises can improve back strength, you need to be cautious if you already have back problems – get some professional advice first.

Training tip

For those moments when you're struggling to do the last few repetitions, try this: Focus all your attention on the muscle that you're using while you do the movement, e.g. your biceps or glutes. Be conscious of really recruiting the muscle group to lift the weights.

Action list

- Find a gym in your area that offers casual strength-training classes at a time to suit you – and give them a try.

- Start off with really light weights at first, but don't be surprised if you feel some muscle soreness the following day or even the second day after a workout. Your body will soon adjust and there'll be fewer muscle aches.

- Try doing a few push-ups from the knees at home (the more you do them, the easier they get).

- If it all seems too daunting, remember this: doing nothing to boost your strength at middle age will only accelerate the muscle loss that's already begun under your skin.

Chapter 3

The energy prescription

*A*erobic (or 'cardio', short for cardiovascular) exercise means any exercise that makes you puff for a minimum of 20 minutes. Aerobic exercise burns up kilojoules (good for weight loss) and makes you fit. This helps your heart and lungs do a better job of delivering oxygen around your body, which makes everything, your brain included, work better.

Being fit makes life easier. It means you can do more without getting tired, including the things you enjoy. And when you sprint for the bus, you're likely to catch it. Exercises that count as aerobic include brisk walking, running or jogging, cardio classes at the gym (including boxing classes and dance classes), cycling, swimming, rowing and tennis.

How much cardio exercise do I need?

Ideally it's good to do three to five sessions of aerobic exercise a week. Try to include a few minutes stretching after each session. Altogether it should add up to at least three or four hours a week, eventually.

If you're not used to exercise, this might seem overwhelming, but you don't have to get to this level overnight – start off small and build up the amount of time you do each week gradually.

To begin with you may be doing only 20–30 minutes a day of walking. If you're not fit, you may find it easier to break this up into two 10–15 minute sessions.

How do I get started?

If you're unused to exercise, walking is always the best place to start. How much you do to begin with depends on how fit you are. But as a general rule, it's best to start off small – say 20 minutes of walking every day, or 30-minutes walking three or four days a week for the first three weeks. The main thing here is to get a regular, achievable habit embedded into your routine – one you can build on.

When you can easily walk for 30 minutes four days a week, you can begin to increase the time so that the walks are longer or more frequent – six or seven days a week.

Choose more than one type of aerobic exercise

There are pros and cons for different kinds of aerobic exercise. It's good to vary the kind of aerobic exercise you do because:

* exercising the same way every day can get monotonous
* doing different exercises works different muscles on different days and challenges your body more
* it also reduces the risk of injury – for instance, you'll reduce the pressure on knee joints if you add in some swimming and cycling instead of just running and walking.

Just because you don't like it at first ...

When you first start exercising, you might not like it. It might seem hard and time consuming. You might wish you were doing something else. That's normal, but give it a chance. The more you start to see and feel results, the more you'll start to like it.

The walking workout

Walking is brilliant exercise – you can do it anywhere, any time and it will help you lose weight, help lower blood pressure and cholesterol, and help prevent diabetes and osteoporosis. Compared to running, there's less impact on your joints and a lower risk of injury – so it's the best way for anyone who's overweight or unused to exercise to get fitter. It's also really easy to build walks into your social or family life.

Once you're used to walking for 30 minutes at a time, making your walk more challenging will improve your fitness and help you lose more weight. You can do this by:

* including some hills and/or steps in your walk
* walking faster
* including bursts of walking – or even jogging – at a faster pace
* walking for longer.

Some experts warn against walking with hand weights, as they can increase the risk of injury. If you need to lose a lot of weight, aim to gradually increase your walking time from 30 minutes to an hour on some days. You can do this in two or three separate sessions through the day – whatever works best within your timetable.

Why walk when you can jog?

The first thing to say here is you don't have to jog – but even if you don't fancy the idea, read this section before you discount it completely.

If the thought 'I could never do that' flashes through your head when a jogger overtakes you in the street, think again. In 2002, a 90-year-old woman completed the London marathon. She'd taken up running at the age of 71. Check out the ages of some of the women who have finished in Australian half-marathon events and you'll see some in their 50s and 60s, as well as Norma Wallett, a 70-something who began running in

Sue Sutton was in her 20s when she began thinking about her future fitness. Could regular walking and yoga help prevent her developing the arthritis and varicose veins that ran in her family? So far, she's winning – at 55 and after two decades of consistent exercise, there's no arthritis, no varicose veins and no weight problems either.

'Walking has never been a chore for me – I've always loved it, partly because it's a mind thing. If you feel down, walking really helps and it gives me energy,' says Sue, who gets up early every morning, in all weather, to walk down to the beach close to her Sydney home before she goes to work. 'I walk for 40 minutes to an hour – not strolls, but fast walks, and on some days I'll have a swim too. Sometimes I'll organise longer walks with friends so we can talk. I don't like the gym but I'm fanatical about walking – I'd go nuts if I didn't walk.'

middle age. This doesn't mean every woman over 45 should be in running shoes, but it proves the point that age isn't always the barrier we think it is.

If you can walk and your knees are okay, the chances are you can run too. You just have to get fit first by regular walking and then start jogging – easing yourself in slowly.

In a time-poor world, running has lots going for it, especially if you do the double act of paid work and parenting. You can run any time, anywhere. It can make you fitter and slimmer faster than walking, and it's easier than you think – you don't need to be good at sport or coordinated to do it. There's no gym membership required and little expense apart from the price of a pair of decent running shoes. And you can begin with baby steps.

I ran my first half-marathon (21.1 kilometres) when I was 48 (and until I started training for it, I'd never run further than four or five kilometres). But when I'd first started running some years before, I didn't think I'd make it around the block, and I hated it. But what I hated even more was the idea of being unfit and having a potbelly. Once you get over the feeling that running is a hard slog (and it takes a few weeks – so hang in there), you can actually begin to find pleasure in it, especially on cool, sparkling mornings. And when the temperature really drops, the pleasure is all in the afterglow – in winter, while everyone else around you is shivering with cold, a run will turn your body's central heating up high. Then there's the buzz – the boost that running gives to your circulation makes you feel like every capillary is humming with energy – and a feeling of running free. Remember that sense of freedom you had when you ran around as a kid? Running can make you feel that again.

When one of my neighbours, 40-year-old Christine, began running recently, her training regime was simple. Run from one telegraph pole to the next, then walk to the next telegraph pole – then run to the next and so on, gradually doing more running segments until she could run for 20 minutes without breaking into a walk. Now she's built up enough endurance to do a 12-kilometre run on occasional weekends with a group of friends.

Compared to walking, running burns more kilojoules and creates an 'afterburn', meaning that your metabolic rate remains higher for a period once you've stopped running, burning a few extra kilojoules.

The downside is that, unless you ease yourself in slowly, you'll soon get sore and disheartened. So it's best to do what Christine did, by alternating bursts of running with walking.

For many women, running's appeal is weight loss, but the health benefits stack up too. Besides reducing the risk of heart disease and diabetes, some studies suggest that vigorous activity like running, cardio classes at the gym and racquet sports may help protect you against breast cancer than gentler activities like walking or golf.

When Sydney GP Jane Givney talks about running, it's like hearing other people praise meditation. It's calming, gives her mind a break, helps her sleep better and makes her more efficient at work, she says – benefits that come not with stillness, but from running for a minimum of five hours a week.

'Running in a group can strengthen the commitment to run – you're more likely to get out of bed if you've arranged to meet someone,' says 45-year-old Louise Heywood, who began running 20 years ago to stay in shape in a job involving constant travel.

'As long as I had my running shoes I could run anywhere in the world,' she adds. 'Like a lot of women, I began running for weight control, then I realised how easy it was and kept on running. If you're consistent, you see improvements in weight loss and fitness quite quickly.' Heywood is a member of the Northside Running Group (NRG), a running club based in St Leonards, open to runners of all levels from beginners to ultra marathons. NRG also offers novice runners a structured eight-week course to learn to run.

'I'd always had this notion I couldn't run,' says Elizabeth Adams, who was 46 when she took up running with NRG. 'I used to feel sick just thinking about the distances some people would run. But if you keep doing it, you can – after six weeks I could run for five kilometres without stopping.'

For 49-year-old Jane, running has been something she can fit around the demands of work and raising five children. 'I can take off by myself when it suits me. I also find it more productive mentally than walking – your mind can process things more freely because nothing else is interacting with you.'

But what about your knees?

Got a problem with your knees? Don't use it as a reason to stay on the couch – doing nothing means you're likely to gain weight, which will only make a knee problem worse. You should get them checked out by an exercise physiologist. While you might think dodgy knees are a sign of arthritis, it could be something else – people with weak core muscles can throw their hips out of place, putting pressure on the knees. An exercise physiologist can identify the problem and map out an exercise program for you.

If your knees are already damaged by a previous knee injury, such as a ligament tear or a torn cartilage, running can increase the risk of developing arthritis. But if you haven't got a problem with your knees and you're scared jogging might give you one, don't be too sure. New research from Monash University in Melbourne suggests short sessions of jogging or aerobics every week may, in fact, be good for knees. The study of 176 women aged from 40 to 67 found that short (around 20 minutes), regular sessions of vigorous activity including tennis, netball and running actually improved knee cartilage – and this in turn may lower the risk of osteoarthritis in the knee, says lead researcher Professor Flavia Cicuttini of the Department of Epidemiology and Preventive Medicine. 'Regular physical activity also protects against muscle weakness, which has been shown to reduce the risk of arthritis,' she says. However, she stresses that the activity sessions were relatively short and that women should still be cautious about taking up running at an older age.

This isn't the only research that says running can actually be good for knees. Researchers at Stanford University in the US followed a group of 538 runners and 423 non-exercisers for almost two decades and found that not only did the runners have less osteoarthritis, but they also had stronger bones as well.

It's thought that female anatomy can make women's knees more injury prone – the trouble starts with a woman's wider pelvis, which makes the thigh bone meet the lower leg bone at an increased angle. The best protection against injury is increasing both the strength of core muscles (to help stabilise your pelvis) and that of your leg muscles. Besides protecting knees, one or two sessions of strength-training a week will also give legs more power and make running easier. It's better for knees if you can run on surfaces with more 'give', such as grass or bush trails rather than bitumen, and don't rely on running alone for a more vigorous cardio workout – mix it up with sessions on an exercise bike or a rowing machine, alternatives that take the pressure off your knees.

What's so hot about running?

Although walking is great exercise, running's advantage is that you improve your cardiovascular fitness faster. By strengthening your heart and lungs, you'll improve your body's oxygen uptake, boosting stamina and reducing fatigue as a result. This is useful stuff. It means you can get through a busy day with energy to spare. If you want to lose weight, you'll do that faster too and get more muscle definition in your legs. And if you're up for it, there's growing evidence that doing something more intense than walking can affect your health. While exercise generally seems to cut women's risk of breast cancer, for instance, research from the long running Nurses' Health Study in the US suggests that more vigorous exercise like jogging could cut the risk even more.

Get the running habit and you've got fitness on a budget. For the price of a pair of running shoes, you have a flexible exercise program you can do anywhere and at a time to suit to you.

* Begin by alternating 60 seconds of running with 90 seconds of walking. Start by running at an easy pace – don't worry about speed at first. Try to run/walk for 20 minutes three times a week – spread these sessions out so you have recovery days in between.
* As you build up endurance, you can gradually increase the running intervals and decrease the walking intervals. Aim to build up to five minutes of running with one minute of walking.
* When you're ready, replace the walking interval with a slow jog instead.
* Gradually increase the intensity of your 20-minute sessions – work on increasing your speed in the running intervals and having shorter recovery intervals of slow jogging. Keep this up until you can run without stopping for 20 minutes.

How do I keep going when I feel like stopping?

If it's breathlessness that makes you want to stop, slow your breathing down and try to focus on the rhythm of your breathing. Often it's your mind that's telling you to stop – try running with smaller steps to push past the feeling of having to stop, even if it feels like you'd move faster if you were walking. Instead of thinking of how much further you have to run, find a landmark a few metres ahead, and once you reach it, find another point and aim for that.

How can I increase my distance?

Build up your running time slowly. Gradually increase the distance of one of your runs by five to ten minutes a week, running at a steady pace, comfortable enough to keep up a conversation. Have a day's rest between runs. Running for 40 to 45 minutes at a stretch is a good long-term goal to aim for, but 30 minutes is good too.

What shoes do I need?

Not your old tennis shoes or cross trainers, but running shoes with good shock absorption to cushion your feet. There should also be a thumb's width gap between your big toe and the end of your shoe. If you're running on the beach, keep your shoes on to avoid injury – running on sand can increase the risk of injuring calves, ankles and Achilles tendons.

Where should I run?

While you can run anywhere, it's best to run on grass or on dirt tracks at least some of the time. Avoid areas of heavy traffic where you'll end up gulping down diesel fumes.

How can I keep cool in hot weather?

Run in the coolest part of the day, preferably in the shade. Skip the Lycra and wear loose cotton shorts and tops or check out sports stores for shorts and tops in fabrics that wick sweat away from your body. Drink plenty of water and wear a hat and sunscreen.

Add a burst of speed. Whether you're walking, running, swimming or pedalling on an exercise bike, vary your pace sometimes so that you're going as fast as you can for a minute or so until you're out of breath. If you're walking, you could break into a jog or a really brisk walk; if you're running, break into a sprint; and if you're pedalling at the gym, go as hard as you can. It's what's called interval training and it used to be an athletes-only technique to improve performance. But it's now considered good for the rest of us too – it gives your workout an edge, helping to improve endurance (meaning you can keep going for longer) and to burn fat.

Take the stairs

Not long ago researchers took a group of sedentary women and got them to change just one thing in their routine: for five days a week over an eight-week period, they had to climb a lot of stairs – not any old stairs, but a public staircase of 199 steps. In the first week they went up the steps once a day, gradually increasing their climbs until they were scaling the stairs five times a day by the eighth. When the eight weeks were up, the women were fitter and their levels of bad LDL cholesterol had dropped.

Stairs are everywhere – they're in our homes, in offices, shopping malls, in parks and on the street – and there are lots of ways you can use them to make you fitter and firmer.

* Stair work is a great butt firmer – especially if you go up the stairs two at a time.
* If there's a choice of stairs or escalator – take the stairs.
* Only an escalator? Run or walk up them.
* Find walking and running routes that incorporate some steps.

Steps can make a shorter workout more effective – try running or walking up and down a set of steps a few times if you're short of time.

Annie Crawford is used to coaching women in their 40s, 50s and even their 60s who once thought they couldn't run – but now know how it feels to pass the finishing line in anything from the nine-kilometre Bridge Run that crosses the Sydney Harbour Bridge each July, to a much longer 21.1 kilometre half-marathon. Annie, 44, an accredited running coach and a distance runner herself, is the brains behind Can Too, the fitness program that Anne Riches and Lee-Anne Carson joined. Many of the women Annie trains have never run before or swum in the ocean – but their age and lack of experience are no barrier, she insists.

'Most people can run as long as they don't have a major injury – we start them off at a slow jog or walking to help them get fit first. What helps them keep going isn't just the personal goal of getting fitter or losing weight, but the fact that they've also made a commitment to help other people.

'In the swimming program we've had women in their 40s who couldn't put their faces under water – and now they're ocean swimming for one or two kilometres,' she says. 'It has a transforming effect on other aspects of their lives too – they say, "Now I feel as if I can do anything."'

As for finding the time to fit in six exercise sessions a week, Annie argues that it can be done. 'For many women, it's easier to make time to exercise in their 40s and 50s than when they were younger and had children who couldn't be left alone. It can be difficult to find time but a lot of it is a mental barrier – if you make it a priority you can do it. I find that once women have finished a ten-week training program with us they don't want to stop exercising so they make the time.'

What other kinds of cardio/aerobic exercise can you do?

SWIMMING

Not as effective for weight loss as walking or running (and doesn't build bone), but has advantages like being gentle on the joints and a great hot weather option. It strengthens and tones all major muscle groups and builds stamina and strength. If you're not a confident swimmer, sign up for a few lessons in summer and improve your swimming for an extra cardio option.

CYCLING

Whether you're on a stationary bike or riding outdoors, cycling is great for boosting fitness and helping with weight loss, and again, it's easy on the joints (though, like swimming, it won't strengthen bones because it's not a weight-bearing exercise). It's a good workout for legs and butt – and a planet-friendly way to get from one place to another.

ROWING, KAYAKING AND CANOEING

These are all terrific workouts for improving fitness, helping with weight loss and strengthening and toning the arms, shoulders, chest and back. You can take to the water or use the rowing machine at the gym.

BOXING

Think boxing isn't for you? Don't be too sure until you've tried it. At the gym where I workout, boxing is one of the most popular classes, and you don't have to look like Hilary Swank to join. It's a great antidote to stress and it combines both cardio and strengthening exercises. Moves like skipping and punching (not a person, but a punching bag or a mitt or pad held by your partner, or even just punching the air) can really get your heart-rate up. There's more than one kind of boxing class – some just involve boxing movements, others are done with a partner where one person holds a mitt or a pad while the other punches it. It's normal to feel clumsy at first because it takes a bit of eye–hand coordination – but you'll improve with practise.

CIRCUIT CLASSES

A circuit class at a gym involves a series of different exercises that include both aerobic and strength-training exercises – e.g. peddling an exercise bike, using a rowing machine, doing some lunges, skipping on the spot, doing bicep curls, stepping up and down on a step. The idea is to do each exercise for a few minutes at a time. Their advantage is that you don't get bored because you're doing so many different things, and you work on different muscle groups. But how effective circuits are for weight loss or fitness depends a lot on each individual class and how hard you work. Some gym chains offer 30-minute women-only circuit classes, which can be a good starting point if you're not used to exercise.

Eating, drinking and exercise

If you're doing something strenuous like running, cycling, swimming laps, or a class at the gym, aim to eat a carbohydrate snack (fruit, wholegrain bread or some yoghurt) about one to two hours beforehand. Don't be tempted to go without to save kilojoules – you'll work better with fuel inside you. But don't eat just before a workout – your body will still be digesting the food and you'll feel uncomfortable. As for fluid, remember you need to drink water before, during and after exercise, especially in hot weather. If you've been exercising strenuously for more than an hour, especially in hot weather, you might need a sports drink. If you want to work out your individual needs for fluid more precisely, you can do this by weighing yourself before and after exercise to see how much fluid you lose. For every kilogram of weight lost, you need to replace one and a half litres of fluid.

Learning to love the gym

There are two kinds of people: those who love the gym and those who loathe it.

But even if you're in the loathe-it camp, there are good reasons to give it a chance – especially if you've never actually tried a gym and simply *think* you won't like it. A gym does have advantages:

◉ It's somewhere to workout when it's uncomfortably cold, hot or wet – good intentions to exercise regularly can be derailed by changeable weather.

- There's music – which can be really motivating and make working out on an exercise bike or doing a class much easier (although it's also one of the things that puts some people off gyms).
- It can be fun! There's a good chance you'll find at least one kind of gym class that you enjoy – yes, you'll get out of breath and it may take a couple of classes before you get all the moves right. But working out to music with other people can be a lot more fun than doing it by yourself.
- Most gyms have a variety of classes you can try so there's a good chance you'll find one that you like. Boxing classes, cardio classes, yoga, Pilates, strength-training, circuit and fitball classes are standard in many gyms. Some have spinning classes (an indoor cycling class on exercise bikes), capoeira (a martial art-cum-dance style), and dance classes like hip hop.
- The advantage of doing different classes is that it stops you getting bored. It also challenges you – your body soon gets used to doing the same kind of exercise and finds it easier to do. This means that after a while you burn up fewer kilojoules doing it. You also learn different ways to use your body to get in shape – and that can only be good for you.

It's time to stand up!

A fit, healthy body doesn't just need structured exercise like a 30-minute walk or a class at the gym, but less time sitting – and this means rethinking how you live every day of the week.

Unless you have a job that keeps you in perpetual motion, you're probably like most of us – glued in a sitting position either in front of a computer, a steering wheel or a TV set for many of your waking hours. This isn't just a recipe for weight gain, there's increasing evidence that too much sitting is bad for us in other ways. When you look at the health of women who exercise regularly, those who spend the most time sitting still have the highest risk of heart disease. Too much sitting can lead to weaker bones, high blood sugar levels and deep vein thrombosis – so be conscious of how much time your butt spends on a seat and figure out how to keep it off for longer.

The 'bottom' line here is that the human body was meant to move – not sit in front of screens. But right now our convenience culture has stolen so much movement from our daily lives that a 30-minute walk or even an hour at the gym can't put back all the movement we've lost, points out Dr Genevieve Healy, a researcher at the School of Population Health at the University of Queensland.

'Although walking or going to the gym do have excellent health benefits, it's often only half an hour or one hour out of a total of 16 waking hours. You can't assume it will compensate for eight to 12 hours of the day spent sitting,' Genevieve says.

But research by Dr Healy, together with the International Diabetes Institute, suggests that clocking up lots of small movements throughout the day, like ironing, washing dishes, putting out the garbage and folding laundry, helps improve both waist measurement and blood sugar levels. She did her research by getting a group of people with an average age of 53 to wear an accelerometer, a gadget similar to a pedometer, but which also measures the intensity at which people exercise. What she found was that the more sedentary people were, the higher their waist measurement and their levels of blood sugar – but the more time they spent on activities rated as light intensity, such as doing the ironing, the healthier their waist measurement and the lower the blood sugar.

Just why lots of small movements help keep blood sugar down isn't yet clear. But the theory is that even small movements make you contract your muscles, and muscles, if you remember, use up blood sugar for fuel. Sitting around, on the other hand, means you're not moving your muscles much, and not using up blood sugar either.

The first time I interviewed exercise scientist Martha Lourey-Bird about weight loss, I thought some of her ideas were, well, nuts. Among her suggestions for accumulating extra activity through the working day was to stand up to answer the phone at work, and to stay standing while you answered the call. Another was to move your rubbish bin further away from the desk so each time you need to use it you have to stand up and move a few steps. How could such teensy movements possibly help anyone shift serious kilos, I wondered?

But while these small steps might be drops in an ocean of lost activity, they really can make a difference. The advice from Martha, a lecturer in the School of Public Health and Community Medicine at the University of NSW and Scientific Adviser to Weight Watchers in Australia, was simply reflecting research that small movements do matter. When researchers at the Mayo Clinic in the US compared the movements of lean people to those of obese people they found that lean people spent an average of two hours a day on small, spontaneous movements like getting up and down, pacing, lifting their arms and generally fidgeting. The extra movement added up to a substantial 1400 kilojoules a day.

To fight the sedentary lifestyles many of us lead, Martha Lourey-Bird says we need to start taking 'long cuts' instead of short cuts.

'We have to create more inconvenience in our lives. Make your work space as inconvenient as possible so that the printer isn't within easy reach, for instance. If it's ten steps there and back to the printer and you do it five times a day, that's 100 steps you wouldn't otherwise have done,' she points out.

Finding extra ways to move may not come easy at first. But once you reset your thinking to look for reasons to move, it will become a habit.

Try and get into a daily routine of calculating how many hours you've spent sitting each day – the more time you've spent in a chair, the more time you need to spend moving around. Or clip on a pedometer and see for yourself how many steps you walk each day – ideally we should be getting 7,500 to 10,000 a day (30 minutes of brisk walking works out at about 4,000 steps).

The irony of sitting down for eight hours or more – as many of us do each day at work – is that it can make you feel so physically tired that all you want to do is sit. But get into the habit of being active and you'll notice that movement perks you up.

Tips for everyday fitness

- Walk or run up an escalator, but never stand still on them. Don't let other people who prefer to stand hold you up – ask them to let you pass.
- Got a spare ten minutes? Go for a walk or think of something active that needs doing. If you're at home, that's likely to mean housework or gardening – tidy something, make the bed, clean the mirrors, water the plants, pull a few weeds, rake some leaves.
- Play with the dog.
- Cleaning the house? Put on a high-energy CD and see how working to music can help you do it faster and enjoy it more – even if you're feeling tired.
- Save energy (the planet's, not yours) and look for ways to do routine chores manually instead of using a gadget that uses power or petrol. You could mow the lawn with a hand mower, or squat down and sweep floors with a dustpan and brush instead of hauling out the vacuum cleaner, or rake leaves instead of using a leaf blower.
- If your job is sedentary, find as many reasons to get up and move as possible – to the water cooler, the loo, to get up and walk to speak to a colleague in the same building instead of phoning or emailing them, or just take a break and walk up and down a few stairs.
- Take a soccer ball and a friend/partner to the park or the beach and kick it around (it can be more fun than running, gets your heart rate up – and seeing a woman kick a football around is no longer an odd sight).
- Skip for a few minutes.
- Hit the floor and do a few push–ups.
- Do some stretches.
- At the supermarket, push your trolley up a ramp rather than taking the lift to get from one level to the next.

Action list

- If you're already walking regularly, look for a route that includes steps or hills to make your walk harder.

- Be conscious of how many hours you spend sitting each day. If there are too many, find extra jobs to do around the house or garden that keep you moving around more.

- Don't worry if you get out of your exercise routine for a week or so – just pick up where you left off.

- Call a friend or a group of friends and arrange to do something this weekend that involves movement – a walk and a cup of coffee is a good start.

Chapter 4

The joy of flex – why middle-aged bodies need to s-t-r-e-t-c-h

A functional, good looking body is fit, strong and flexible. Building some stretching into your fitness routine is another way of tackling the invisible stiffening and tightening that goes on under your skin to make you look older on the outside. Muscles tend to get shorter and stiffer as you get older, and stretching helps counteract this. It also helps you maintain the resilience of connective tissue; this means your tendons and ligaments, as well as the thin layer of tissue (called fascia) that wraps groups of muscle fibre together within muscles, and encases each muscle on the outside. Ageing, poor posture and inactivity can tighten the fascia and restrict your movement

Being supple is useful – it lets you bend, reach, stretch and twist more easily, and by increasing your range of movement you'll improve your balance too. Supple is also a good look. It's the opposite of stiff, and bodies that are supple and move easily look so much younger than bodies that move stiffly. Does this mean you have to somehow fit in yoga and Pilates sessions *and* work on your cardio fitness and muscle strength? Not necessarily. There are lots of ways of building stretching into your routine. If there's time to fit in a session of yoga and Pilates, that's perfect – doing either of these activities regularly also teaches you stretches that you can do at home. But if you don't have time to fit in a class, be sure to do some stretching after each workout and try to find other times to fit in a few stretches.

You can do stretches any time – at your desk or in front of TV – but

'I hear people say, "Yoga can make you flexible but it doesn't get you fit",' says Wendy Guest, 50, a journalist who is now training to become a yoga teacher. 'Flexibility, it seems, is the second cousin to fitness – that is, until you twist your back reaching for your handbag behind you in the car, or find it too hard to get down and tie your shoes. To me, flexibility is the most important goal as I get older. At 50 I am more flexible than I was at 40. At 60 I'll be more flexible than I am today. I can get fit by walking, rowing or riding a bike. Increasing my flexibility gently and daily is a gift I'm giving my body for its future.'

it's important to stretch after exercise when your muscles are warmer, more flexible and easier to stretch.

Should I stretch before I workout?

Most experts say there's no need. What's more important is to warm-up your muscles for a few minutes by doing a kind of gentle rehearsal of the activity you're about to do – for example, walking before you start your run, or warming up for strength-training by doing some of the movements you do when you lift weights, only with lighter weights or using no weights.

Will Pilates or yoga help me lose weight too?

As well as improving flexibility, both yoga and Pilates can help increase strength – though they won't tone muscle and shape your body in the same way as strength-training can. As for weight loss, only faster forms of yoga that get your heart rate up are likely to help you burn kilojoules. Although one study of overweight middle-aged people found that those who did yoga lost a few kilos compared to those who did nothing, the researchers believed this had more to do with the fact that the yoga practitioners tended to eat healthier and take better care of themselves. In other words, except for perhaps power yoga, a westernised version of Ashtanga yoga, don't expect either yoga or Pilates to help with weight loss in the same ways that aerobic exercise, such as regular walking, jogging or gym classes do.

But while they're no substitute for cardio exercise and strength-training, for anyone who's really inactive, yoga and Pilates can be a stepping stone to becoming more active and building exercise into your week. If you find the gym intimidating, one way of overcoming this might be to start by joining a yoga or Pilates class at the gym rather than a cardio or strength class.

Yoga, Pilates and other stretch classes can be effective stressbusters too – and reducing stress can be another way of taming hot flushes. Even if you don't plan to do yoga or Pilates regularly, it's worth trying out a few classes to pick up some exercises you can build into your own routine.

What Pilates can do for you

Pilates' slow movements can ease you into becoming more active and, if you're already exercising, Pilates is a great add-on for boosting flexibility in a way that walking, running or cardio classes at the gym can't do.

Pilates is a form of exercise using slow, controlled exercises done on a mat or on special equipment to strengthen and lengthen muscles and improve posture, flexibility and balance. While it won't shed kilos, it will make you more toned and give you a longer, leaner look. It's also an antidote to sedentary 21st-century living. Besides becoming less active, we've become more limited in our range of movements – there's no need to do the same amount of twisting, reaching or bending that people once did before appliances came along to do it all for us.

If you spend much of your week sitting in front of a keyboard or a steering wheel, you force your spinal muscles to work overtime by under-using the deepest layer of abdominal muscles that are meant to hold you up – this is the *transversus abdominis* (TA muscle for short) that wraps around your body like a corset between your ribs and hips. Pilates can help retrain this muscle – the key is to visualise your pelvic floor as a trampoline suspended between your tail bone at the back, your pubic bone at the front and your hip bones at either side. Imagine there's a string in the middle of the trampoline, and try to draw it upwards – this helps you engage the muscles of your lower abs. Now imagine you're drawing your navel into your spine. Engaging these deep abdominals is part of all Pilates exercises, but it's also a movement you can take into everyday life.

It should be the first thing you do when you bend your knees to lift a heavy load because it takes the stress off your back. If you practise 'navel to spine' some of the time while sitting or walking, it will improve your posture and protect your lower back.

While you might not break a sweat doing Pilates, it can be a challenging workout because the moves are so precise you have to really think about what you're doing. But it's this mental focus that can be such a good stressbuster because it empties your head of everything else. You also have to learn to breathe correctly – breathing deeply gets more oxygen to your muscles so you stretch more easily.

Pilates can make a difference after just one workout – as if someone has gently rearranged your body and nudged every muscle and bone into its rightful place. One of the most common things people say when they start Pilates is 'I watch how I sit now'. This new awareness, along with the strengthening of your postural muscles, helps you improve your posture without having to think about it.

Some Pilates classes involve only floor exercises, while others combine floor work with Pilates machines. Either way, the movements are similar – the difference is that the machines make it easier to get the moves right and also help you stretch further than you thought possible. Because workouts on machines are done in small groups – generally in small studios rather than gyms – the exercises can be tailored to your individual needs.

You can choose either mat work or machines – or combine both. If you have an injury, mat work isn't for you. Start with a one-to-one session to begin with, and then a small group.

The benefits of yoga

Yoga is a mind–body workout. Similar to Pilates, the mental focus on the different movements can do a good job of stilling your mind. Like Pilates it also helps you learn to increase your core strength. Although the term core stability sounds new, the same concept of strengthening the deep band of muscle that swaddles the body below the navel has been part of many yoga styles for thousands of years. Like Pilates, yoga's postures counteract the muscle weakness and inflexibility that come from hours of inactivity slouched at our desks or behind a steering wheel, and help to put back some of the natural twisting and bending we did in the days before we became chairbound.

'At a yoga class in my 40s I met a woman who was probably in her 60s and amazingly flexible. When she did an intense seated forward bend called *paschimotanasana*, she folded into a perfect hinge at the hips, flattening her stomach to her thighs with her legs and back still beautifully long and straight. It sounds simple to sit on the floor and fold forward with a flat back – but try it!' says Wendy Guest. Many of us can get our noses somewhere near our knees by hunching our spine over, but to fold like this 60-year-old takes a lot of openness and flexibility in the hips and length in the hamstrings. My *paschimotanasana* is still a distance from her pose, but it's moving in the right direction – and each small increment of additional and comfortable stretch I feel gives me enormous pleasure.'

No time for yoga or Pilates?

Try to stretch three to five times a week for ten minutes or so. You can do stretches any time – at work or in front of the TV at home, but, ideally, do them after a workout. A class at the gym will include stretches at the end of the workout, and a strength-training class will also include stretches after each individual exercise as well. The reason for stretching after an exercise is that muscles stretch more easily when they're 'warm'

from moving around – stretching muscles without warming them up
first can cause an injury. If you do stretches without doing a workout
first, you still need to warm up by moving around for a few minutes. Find
opportunities to stretch throughout the day – take a break from your
desk to do a few stretches. Or do what I do – if you're stuck with nothing
to do for a few minutes, or you're trapped in a supermarket queue, sneak
in a few discreet standing stretches like the hamstring stretch.

Tips for stretching

- Stretching should never cause pain, especially joint pain. Hold a
  stretch at what's called the stretch threshold – when you can feel
  a 'pull' but not pain. If it hurts, you're stretching too far, and you
  need to reduce the stretch until it doesn't hurt.
- Stretching should be a smooth, slow movement – don't bounce
  or jerk when you stretch.
- Hold each stretch for 30 to 60 seconds.
- Remember to relax and keep breathing while you stretch.
- Don't 'lock' your joints into a dead straight position when you
  straighten them during a stretch. Your arms and legs should be
  straight when you stretch them, but with a little bend in your joints.

Some simple stretches

HAMSTRING STRETCH

You should feel this stretch along the back of your thigh. Lie on your
back with your left knee bent and foot flat on the floor. Raise your right
leg in the air and put your hands behind your calf or thigh. Then bring
your knee in towards your chest, slowly straightening your leg so the
sole of your foot is facing up to the ceiling. Try to pull your leg in as close
to your body as possible. Repeat on the other side.

SHOULDER STRETCH

To help keep shoulders flexible, bring your left arm across your body and hold it with your right arm, either above or below the elbow. Repeat on the other side.

LOWER BACK STRETCH

Lie on your back with your arms outstretched. Bend your left knee at 90°. Put your right hand on your left thigh and pull your bent left knee over the right leg. Keeping your head on the floor, turn to look towards your outstretched left arm. Pull your bent left knee towards the floor, keeping your shoulders flat on the floor. Repeat on the other side.

UPPER BACK STRETCH

Put your hands together in front of you and then push them out away from you, keeping your hands clasped so you round out your upper back. You should feel the stretch between your shoulder blades.

Action list

- Look for casual Pilates or yoga classes in your area. Try a few sessions to learn more about stretching.

- Take advantage of warmed-up muscles after a walk, run or other exercise and spend a few minutes stretching.

- Remember to practise 'navel to spine' while you're sitting or walking to improve your posture and protect your lower back.

- Find a high shelf and reach up to touch it with both hands. Feel the s-t-re-tch through your legs, back, shoulders and arms. Think how good it feels to stretch that far – and how frustrating it would be if you couldn't. Nurture your flexibility.

Part Two
Diet and lifestyle

Chapter 5

Preventing midlife kilo creep

*T*here are good reasons for a diet makeover at 40+. Besides helping prevent midlife weight gain, better eating habits (and more exercise) can help with a clutch of other health issues, such as reducing the risk of chronic disease and improving some symptoms of menopause too. But, just as there are no unicorns and no tooth fairies, there are no short cuts to successful weight loss – and any program claiming rapid loss of kilos should set alarm bells ringing. The only thing you're likely to lose in a hurry is money. Kilos that drop off fast have a habit of creeping back on, while those that come off slowly are more likely to stay off. Extra weight doesn't grow on your body overnight, it creeps on slowly over time, and peeling it off permanently also takes time.

This may not be what you want to hear, but accepting it makes it easier to stay focused on what really works – making lasting changes to how you eat, not a few weeks of panic dieting in spring to off-load winter flab.

Let's begin by looking at some of the not-so-obvious causes that make it easier to gain weight at midlife – and harder to lose it.

Why the 21st century is making us fatter

Any woman trying to cope with the shape-shifting effects of menopause today is doing it tougher than her mother and grandmother did at the same age. We're now living in a time when controlling weight is harder than it's ever been before. There's been a big change in the way we live in the last three decades, and it's affecting our size – especially at midlife.

For starters, we live in a crazy society where the kind of food that feeds a weight problem is more aggressively promoted than healthier stuff that would help keep us lean. When was the last time you saw a TV ad urging you to eat more fresh broccoli or Chinese greens – or a billboard declaring that the average woman needs to take about 3000 steps to use up the kilojoules in a small 30-gram packet of chips?

We've also lost control of what we eat, relying more on processed convenience food or takeaway to which someone else has added ingredients like cheap, unhealthy fats, salt and sugar that do no favours to our health or our waistline. And it's not just the kilojoule content of some of these foods that's causing our weight problems, but often their flavours or their textures. It's so easy to overeat food that's either very sweet or very salty, as many processed foods are. These flavours can seduce your tastebuds, but without delivering decent nutrition. The same goes for food that's over refined – think instant noodles, soft white bread and cakes. They slip down with so little chewing that it's easy to eat too much. When was the last time you ate too many pears?

While kilojoule-dense food is available around the clock, it's becoming harder to get even minimal amounts of exercise to help chew up these kilojoules before they're stored as fat – and lack of time is part of the problem. Compared to their grandmothers, women in their 40s now are more likely to be working the double shift of a day job and meeting the needs of a family at night.

'I'm starting to feel as if my body's now on some slippery slope – it seems to be harder to stay in shape, yet it's so difficult to find the time to do anything about it,' says a 44-year-old Canberra friend with a full-time job in the public service and two children. 'It's great if I can get to the gym twice a week after work – but then I've still got dinner to make and I worry that I'm neglecting the kids if I'm not home straight after work.'

Even when children turn into teenagers technically capable of taking more care of themselves, a woman's workload may not lighten up. If the kids themselves are overstretched with study and extra activities, parents

– often mothers – are the ones taking up the slack, providing support and driving them around.

When women in their late 40s come to Sheryl Macrow-Cain for help to lose weight or get fitter, she asks them how much time they have for themselves during the week. The answer is often no time at all.

'I've been working as a personal trainer for ten years and in that time I've seen women getting fatter. They're also more likely to be on medication for depression or because their blood pressure and cholesterol levels are too high,' she adds. 'They often don't have time to cook healthy meals and are relying on processed food.'

For some women, pressure of full-time work and the time squeeze that goes with it can affect their weight. Another interesting difference between the weight gainers and the non-gainers in the Women's Health Australia Survey mentioned earlier was that weight gainers were more likely to work full-time and report that being under time pressure resulted in a higher kilojoule intake. Eating healthily can be one of the first casualties of too much to do and too little time – decisions about what to eat get left to the last minute, making it tempting to opt for more takeaway or convenience food.

But the irony of 21st-century living is that, while our lives have sped up, our bodies have slowed down. Physically we're becoming more and more passive as tightening schedules squeeze out time for regular exercise. We're relying more heavily on appliances or other people to do the physical activities previous generations did themselves. Outsourcing chores like lawn mowing or car washing and using technology to take us from one floor to the next is stealing chunks of kilojoule-burning movement from our lives – and that's not counting the time spent travelling by car that we once did on foot or bicycle, nor the computers that have shrunk so much physical activity down to movements made with our fingers. Who needs to walk across a room to file a document when a couple of mouse clicks can do it for you?

And does anyone remember school assignments pre-internet, and

'I find ageing less stressful because my body hasn't really changed over the years,' says Bev Hadgraft, a 48-year-old Sydney writer. 'I think it's a hassle to gain weight – you only have to lose it, so I've always tried to keep in shape and be proactive about my health. I've read a lot about how the body deteriorates with age and I'm doing everything I can to counteract it.'

'Everything' includes eating a lot of vegetables and fruit, a little fish and chicken, but no meat. Breakfast is muesli with fruit, yoghurt and soy milk, lunch is usually a healthy sandwich of some kind or a vegetable soup; dinner might be a stir fry or a salad. Along with this is an average of one hour's exercise a day – it could be cycling, running, surfing or strength-training.

'I'm doing more strength-training because I know it will keep me strong as I get older. It makes me feel more confident about the future – I want to be able to travel, and I don't want to have to worry that I can't walk very far or that I can't get into a kayak.'

how helping kids research anything from the Gold Rush to Genghis Khan meant moving major muscle groups to go to the local library? Now we let Wikipedia do the walking and there's no need to leave our chairs. It's easier than ever to slide into more sedentary habits as we get older – and the less active we get, the less attractive exercise becomes. No wonder our waistlines are blowing out and big girls' clothes are getting bigger … and bigger.

With menopause breathing down your neck, it's time to audit your eating – not just to iron out belly fat, but to fend off health problems that have more to do with habits than age. Sticking to a healthy weight is *the* most important factor for women in avoiding problems like heart disease, diabetes and arthritis, according to the Women's Health Australia Survey. Excess weight slows you down, sapping your physical energy and causing more wear and tear on joints, especially in the knees, which bear so much of your weight. This can have an effect that's, quite literally, crippling, and this extra weight increases the risk of arthritis. As you gain weight, your knees hurt more and, as a result, you move less. This leads to further weight gain and the unhealthy cycle continues.

There's an extra pay-off for eating better and moving more at menopause – along with whittling your waist, it can help preserve bone and possibly your mind too. There's good evidence that what we eat and how much we move can influence our chances of developing dementia as we get older.

Check the statements below – how many describe the way you eat and shop?

Rate your plate.

* When I go shopping it's to buy mainly fresh and unprocessed foods.
* I rarely eat fast food.
* The carbs I eat are mostly 'smart carbs', like wholegrain or sourdough bread, oats or barley.
* I eat meals that include legumes a couple of times a week.
* Between meals I'll nibble on fruit and nuts – I rarely eat snack foods.
* When I open the fridge door I can see lots of vegetables.
* When I look at what I'm eating for dinner, most of my plate is filled with different coloured plant foods.
* I make an effort to get enough calcium in my diet either through low fat dairy products and/or non-dairy foods like almonds, leafy greens and calcium-enriched soy milk.
* When I eat meat and poultry it's lean and in modest amounts.
* I can't remember the last time I ate sausages.
* I avoid processed meats like ham, bacon and salami.
* Sometimes I'll eat a rich dessert or have a good piece of cake with coffee – but it's a treat, not a regular thing.

- I rarely snack on biscuits.
- I eat fish at least twice a week.
- I eat breakfast every day.
- If I need a drink, I'll have water rather than a soft drink.
- I try to keep my sodium intake low.

If most of these statements apply to you, you're on track – if not, get ready to make some changes.

What's the best way to lose fat?

Before you start any weight-loss plan, get one thing clear – it's not just weight you want to lose, but fat. Here are three important points to remember:

 The loss of body fat (not the loss of fluid and muscle that can also show up as weight loss on the scales) is what improves your health and helps keep weight off in the long term. When weight loss is rapid, it might be because you're losing fluid and muscle tissue as well as fat. Losing muscle is like shooting yourself in the foot – it only makes your body less efficient at burning kilojoules.

 When a weight loss program claims people can lose 17 kg in five weeks, you can bet that amount of weight loss couldn't possibly be all fat. Yet if weight loss is slower, around half a kilo a week or two kilos a month, the more likely it is that you're losing fat – and, better still, the more likely it is that the weight loss will be sustainable.

Don't get obsessed with the numbers on the scales, especially if you've added in strength-training to your routine. Just because the scales don't show much weight loss, doesn't mean you're not losing fat. The combination of eating healthier and exercising more means you'll lose fat but gain muscle. Because muscle is denser than fat, it weighs more. A better way to tell how you're doing is to check your waist measurement or how your clothes fit.

There's lots of different ways of eating that can help you shift weight – you could follow a higher protein diet such as the CSIRO Diet, join Weight Watchers, switch to vegetarian eating, or follow a low GI diet – there's research that says they can all help take the kilos off. But there are questions to ask when you're choosing a way of eating to help you lose weight and keep it off, especially when you're over 40, such as:

- Will this diet do more than drop my dress size? Can it also protect my long-term health?
- Does it include a wide variety of foods so I can be sure of getting a broad mix of different nutrients?
- Can I stick with this way of eating long-term, not just for a few weeks?

Making sense of the carbs versus protein debate

Sometimes it seems like we're involved in a tug of war between two opposing diet tribes. On one side, there are the protein warriors urging us to eat like our hunter–gatherer ancestors – more animal protein and fewer carbohydrates. And in the carb camp, the supporters of low GI carbs – the slow-burning carbohydrate foods that help keep blood sugar levels more even. So, which eating style works best for weight loss? The answer, unfortunately, is not as simple as that. Both can be effective. But which one will also keep you healthier as you reach midlife, when the risks of heart disease, diabetes and cancer start to rise?

At this stage there's not enough research to give a firm answer either way, but some studies suggest that diets high in animal protein also increase LDL cholesterol. This raises questions about their effects on health in the long term. On the other hand, we do know that it's good to eat some healthy carbs – think dense wholegrain breads, barley, rolled oats and legumes. These quality carbs, high in cholesterol-lowering fibre and nutrients, are kind to the heart and gut. They're also menopause-friendly too – wholegrains, especially wholegrain rye, also contain lignans – weak plant oestrogens that may help improve some symptoms of menopause.

The argument for a diet higher in animal protein and lower in carbs is that, for many people, it's easier to stick with, it fills you up so you're not always snacking and it provides important nutrients like iron and zinc, which many women are low in. People's metabolisms differ, so it is sometimes hard to predict how their bodies will handle carbs. Some of us can eat lots and burn them up, while others tend to put on weight and do better on a diet that's lower in carbs rather than one that just cuts kilojoules across the board (though this doesn't mean anyone should be wiping carbohydrates from their diet entirely).

What about the idea that a diet high in animal protein is healthier because it's what our hunter–gatherer ancestors evolved to eat? The flaw in this argument is that the meat our ancestors ate was different to what's on special at the supermarket. It didn't come from animals that spent their lives standing around eating in paddocks or feed lots – it came from leaner wild game, often on the run from predators. This means it would have had a healthier fat profile – less saturated fat and more of the healthier polyunsaturated and monounsaturated fats.

Another issue is the link between eating a lot of red meat and cancer. Recent research from the World Cancer Research Fund suggests that a diet high in meat – meaning more than 500 g (cooked weight) of red meat a week – can increase the risk of some cancers, including bowel cancer.

That said, a way of eating that's higher in protein doesn't have to include lots of red meat – fish and lean poultry are other good protein sources. The bottom line is that a healthy weight loss plan for a woman at menopause needs both carbs and protein, preferably together at each meal. They're a good combination for keeping you full and less tempted to snack too much. The important thing is to be choosy about which carbs and what kind of protein.

Smart rules to eat by

STACK YOUR PLATE WITH PLANTS

At least two thirds of the food on your plate should be made up of a variety of plant foods, mostly a mix of different vegetables, and with some whole grains, pasta or starchy veg like potato or sweet potato too. The remainder should be some kind of lean protein (fish, skinless poultry, lean meat, eggs, reduced fat dairy food, or plant protein like nuts, legumes or tofu). This isn't just a recipe for weight loss – eating more of the right kind of plant foods may help prevent chronic disease as well. It might even preserve muscle – recent studies suggest that a diet rich in potassium from vegetables and fruit may help us preserve muscle mass as we get older. As far as weight is concerned, vegetables are lower in kilojoules (we're not including fries here!) and often take time to chew. They also tend to be higher in fibre, which helps fill you up. More vegetables and some wholegrains on your plate also leave less room for other foods that are higher in kilojoules.

OPEN FEWER PACKETS OF PROCESSED FOOD

Eat more fresh food, or whole food, meaning food that's as close as possible to the way nature intended it, and less processed food. The problem with much processed food isn't just that it's less nutritious and often loaded with sodium, additives and preservatives, but because it often has less fibre, softer textures and more intense, more-ish flavours that make it easy to eat too much.

EAT BREAKFAST – WHEN YOU'RE READY

In studies of people who lose weight and keep it off, eating breakfast shows up consistently as one of the habits they have in common. While it seems counter-intuitive that eating something helps you lose weight, the theory is that, with a healthy breakfast inside you, you're less likely to get hungry later on and snack on junk. But the reality is that sometimes there's no time to eat breakfast, or you don't feel like food first thing – the morning rush to get out of the house can be enough to shut down digestion.

While eating breakfast is important, when you eat it isn't. You can eat it at work or on the way. The solution is forward planning – spend a few minutes the night before making a portable breakfast to eat either on the way to work or when you arrive. This way you're not starting work on an empty stomach – something that can set you up for eating too many kilojoules later on. It's also an easy way of packing in important nutrients – calcium, protein and the heart-friendly fibre that a healthy 40- or 50-something woman needs.

For a breakfast that helps you go the distance, include a good carb (traditional oats, dense, grainy bread or wholegrain breakfast cereal) with protein, such as low fat yoghurt, milk or soy milk, an egg, baked beans, nuts or seeds, and try to include some fresh or dried fruit. With this combination, you're less likely to need sugar hits through the day.

Fast breakfast combinations include:

* untoasted muesli with low fat natural yoghurt and fresh fruit
* soy and linseed, pumpernickel or rye bread toast spread with low fat ricotta and berries
* fruit smoothie with low fat yoghurt and/or soymilk and toasted wholegrain bread.

If you have more time:

* a small bowl of porridge with low fat milk – stir in some sliced banana, dates, grated apple or finely chopped pear as it cooks
* a poached egg, or baked beans on toast.

Portable breakfasts:

* carton of low fat yogurt with a handful of dried fruit and nuts or seeds
* soy and linseed bread with a hard-boiled egg and small piece of fruit
* a container of untoasted muesli mixed with low fat yoghurt or buttermilk, and berries or grapes.

EAT GOOD CARBS – NOT NO CARBS

You know something's wrong when the (skinny) woman ordering dinner at the next table asks anxiously – does veal schnitzel have carbs in it? Or when your girlfriend offers you the hunk of sourdough bread that comes with her soup because 'I'm dieting and keeping off carbs', then orders sticky date pudding with cream for dessert.

Carbohydrates have been given a bad reputation recently – and some of them really deserve it: soft drinks, doughnuts, mass-produced biscuits and cakes, breakfast cereals that are low in fibre and high in sugar and salt should be on anyone's hit list. Even if weight's not an issue, these foods deliver so little nutrition for so many kilojoules that they're just not worth eating. Wholegrain cereals, vegetables, legumes and fruit, on the other hand – all of them carbohydrates – have a lot going for them, including fibre and a load of other nutrients that help prevent heart disease, diabetes and possibly some cancers.

This doesn't mean bingeing on carbs though – it means eating moderate amounts and being choosy about which ones you eat. If my friend had opted for the hunk of sourdough bread (about 728 kJ without butter), she wouldn't have had room for the pud (around 2300 kJ, if you include the cream), saving herself nearly 1600 kilojoules.

If you need to lose weight, it's okay to eat fewer carbs, but don't wipe them out of your diet. Do that and you'll miss out on important nutrients, says Dr Clare Collins, Associate Professor in Nutrition and Dietetics at the University of Newcastle. Although you'll lose weight rapidly, this loss will be water, not fat. The reason? Your muscles act like a fuel tank storing reserves of carbohydrate – called glycogen – that is stored with water. If your diet is too low in carbs, your body will use up these reserves. Despite the fact that the result will show up as weight loss on the scales, what you've lost is only the water, that was stored with the glycogen.

A smarter approach is to eat smaller servings of quality carbs, including wholegrains – the bulkier grains that humans used to eat before industrial food processing came along and made carbohydrates softer and more refined.

Just how many serves is best for weight loss depends on what works for you – some dietitians suggest four serves a day is a reasonable amount, others suggest six.

How much is a single serve of carbs?

One serve =

* ½ cup cooked grains (rice, bulgur, traditional oats, quinoa, barley, pasta)
* a slice wholegrain bread (as grainy as possible, preferably with seeds added)
* ½ cup of a starchy vegetable – potato, sweet potato or legumes
* 1 cup rolled oats.

Should you avoid eating carbs after 6pm if you want to lose weight? There are lots of different versions of this 'no carbs in the evening' rule, ranging from 'no carbs after 5 pm' to 'no carbs after 7 pm'. Although there's no reason to bar carbohydrates in the evening, there's a case for being choosy about the *type* of carbs you eat and how much. If you want to lose weight, then drinking alcohol and eating a pile of pasta or dessert at a time of day when you're inactive won't help. But having a small portion of brown rice or a small potato, with plenty of vegetables and some lean protein, is fine.

Get to know the difference between low GI and high GI carbs.

Carbs that create a slower, smaller rise in blood sugar – like oats and dense wholegrain breads – are generally healthier in the long term than those that make it shoot up rapidly e.g. cake or biscuits. What the Glycaemic Index (GI) does is to rank foods containing carbs according to how they affect your blood sugar. If they make it rise quickly, they're ranked as a high GI food. Low GI foods, on the other hand, are those that take longer to digest, causing a lower more gradual rise in blood sugar.

Because you digest them more slowly, many low GI carbs are good for appetite control – they make you feel fuller for longer, so you're less likely to overeat or keep grazing between meals.

- Low GI foods have a GI of less than 55
- Medium GI foods have a GI of between 56 and 69
- High GI foods have a GI of more than 70.

EAT SOME LEAN PROTEIN AT EVERY MEAL

Protein will help you feel full and also helps you preserve muscle, and that's important for any 40- or 50-something woman who wants to lose weight. The recommended daily intake (RDI) for adults in Australia is about one gram of protein per kilo of body weight a day. The table opposite gives you an idea of how much protein you get from different foods.

Although red meat has a reputation for being 'fattening', it's quite the opposite – lean meat can help you lose weight. But is it healthy? That depends on what kind of meat you eat and how much. There's good advice in Australia's official nutrition bible, *The Dietary Guidelines for Adults in Australia*, which suggests eating surprisingly small amounts of red meat – just 65-100 g of cooked red meat (about the size of the palm of your hand), three or four times a week. (Remember that sausages and salami don't count as lean meat.)

If you don't eat red meat, the protein alternatives are:

* 65–100 g cooked chicken
* 80–120 g cooked fish fillet
* 2 small eggs
* ½ cup cooked beans, lentils, chickpeas, split peas, dried or canned beans
* ⅓ cup nuts

How much protein is that?*

Food	Protein
120 g steamed fish fillet	29 g
100 g lean beef	30 g
½ chicken breast	26 g
100 g canned salmon or tuna	22 g
1 egg	6 g
6 large prawns	14 g
125 g cottage cheese	15.5 g
20 g slice of cheese	5 g
200 g yoghurt	11 g
250 ml low fat milk	9.8 g
2 slices wholegrain bread	8–12 g (breads with more seeds and soy are higher in protein)
60 g muesli	7 g

* Values are approximate.

EAT HEALTHIER FATS

Science is challenging the idea, etched on our brains throughout the 1980s and 1990s, that eating fat makes you fat. While all fats have the same number of kilojoules – around 38 kJ per gram – they may not all have the same effect on your weight. Too much saturated fat (mainly in food from animals, including dairy products, manufactured cakes, biscuits and in coconut milk) can expand your waistline, but there's some evidence that people who eat healthy fats from nuts, seeds, avocado, olive oil and oily fish, for instance, tend to pack less fat around the waist compared to those who eat a high level of saturated fat. Eating these healthier fats is good for you in other ways: the type of fat you spread on toast or drizzle on a salad may decrease the risk of arthritis and depression, as well as heart disease. That's why many experts suggest eating a variety of fats and eating them in their food form – think oily fish, nuts, seeds and avocado. That way we get other nutrients in the food we don't get from the oil alone.

A wider mix of fats also makes for a healthier balance of two important fats in our diet – omega-6 and omega-3 fats. Both are 'good' polyunsaturated fats – omega-6 fats are in corn, safflower or sunflower oil, while omega-3 fats are in oily fish, walnuts, flax seed (linseed), soybeans and some dark leafy greens. But in a typical Western diet, the balance of these fats is out of whack – we're eating too few omega-3 fats and too many omega-6 fats mainly because our diets have been overloaded with omega-6 fats in the form of cooking oils and margarines and in many processed foods that contain these foods. Research now suggests that this imbalance contributes to health problems including arthritis, depression and the hidden inflammation that can increase the risk of heart disease and other problems.

But a better balance of these fats, created by eating more fish, walnuts, flaxseed and leafy greens, for example, may prevent heart disease and reduce psoriasis, rheumatoid arthritis, depression and possibly asthma. Omega-3 fats are heart-friendly, raising levels of 'good' cholesterol and helping prevent clotting.

But if you want to lose weight, how do you eat them without adding too many kilojoules to your diet?

* *Take control of how much and what kind of fat you eat* by eating more fresh wholefoods and fewer processed foods (which often contain the kind of fat you want to avoid, e.g. saturated fat, trans fats, as well as too much omega-6 polyunsaturated fat). Eating less processed food means *you* decide how much fat is used in a dish – not the manufacturer.

* *Use small amounts of olive oil for cooking.* Olive oil is a good choice – it's a monounsaturated fat which doesn't contribute any extra omega-6 fats to the diet. Canola is okay too – it contains some omega-3 fats – but it has less flavour and fewer antioxidants than olive oil.

* *Use olive oil spray* for roasting vegetables or for toasting bread in the oven – you use less fat.

* *Use cold pressed extra virgin olive oil* in salad dressings (cold pressed has the most antioxidants). With its good flavour, a little goes a long way.

* *It's okay to eat nuts.* They are high in kilojoules but the trick is (a) not to eat them mindlessly by the bowlful, and (b) eat them instead of, not as well as, other foods. In other words, don't snack on corn chips *and* nuts – just have small handful of nuts. Or swap nuts for meat one night a week. They're a good source of protein that needs little preparation in meals, for example, cashews or pistachios stir fried with ginger and Chinese greens. Or toss some walnuts into a salad instead of croutons or cheese. According to research, nut eaters are no heavier than anyone else.

* *Avoid using margarines made from safflower and sunflower oil.* So what should you put on bread? Maybe nothing – make a sandwich with a moist filling and you don't actually need a spread. Or try mashed avocado, low fat ricotta, hummus or bread toasted in the oven with a little olive oil sprayed on.

* *Linseed (flaxseed) contains omega-3 fats.* A tablespoon adds texture to muesli (it's good in home-baked cakes and muffins too). Flaxseed might also improve menopause symptoms – a small US study by the Mayo Clinic has suggested that 40 grams daily can reduce hot flushes, but this research is not yet conclusive. Sandra Villella, naturopath with The Jean Hailes Foundation for Women's Health in Melbourne, recommends two dessertspoons of flaxseed daily. There's some evidence that this can help reduce vaginal dryness around menopause, she says. Stick to ground linseeds (you digest them better than whole linseed), and it's best to buy them whole and grind them yourself in a coffee grinder, and then store them in the fridge.

EAT YOUR KILOJOULES – DON'T DRINK THEM

Most of us wouldn't eat our way through four apples in one go – but if we did it would take time to get through them and, thanks to all the chewing and the 13 grams of fibre they contain, we'd feel very full. But a large 650 ml carton of apple juice takes a couple of minutes to gulp down, has no fibre and delivers 1300 kilojoules – the equivalent of three slices of toast and butter – without filling you up. This doesn't mean juices are bad – they're packed with vitamins, minerals and antioxidants. Some juices, including dark grape juice and cloudy apple juice (the cloudy juice contains the peel), are especially antioxidant rich. But if weight loss is your goal, you need to cut kilojoules and increase your fibre intake, so it makes sense to drink water to quench your thirst and to eat an apple or a few grapes instead. Or you could drink water with a splash of juice. If you're ordering juice from a juice bar – or using the juicer at home – juice made with vegetables and fruit, rather than fruit alone, will have fewer kilojoules.

KEEP EATING HEALTHILY AT WEEKENDS

While everyone needs a treat sometimes, the idea that it's okay to indulge over the weekend as long as you eat healthily throughout the week is unlikely to keep the weight off. There are only seven days in a week, and the weekend includes two of them. That's plenty of time to eat too many kilojoules. Extra food and alcohol eaten over Friday night, Saturday and Sunday can add a lot of extra kilojoules. Successful losers take a consistent approach to food, which includes eating sensibly at weekends, as well as during the week.

DON'T LET YOURSELF GET TOO HUNGRY

Allowing yourself to get so famished you'll fall on anything as long as it kills the hunger pangs can stoke a weight problem. If you know you'll get hungry between meals and won't have access to healthy food, be proactive – carry fruit and nuts with you. It makes it easier to resist high kilojoule food like chocolate, muffins, biscuits and chips. Go too long without eating and you're likely to overeat when you do finally get food – raging hunger can make you eat so fast that you don't give your stomach time to register that it's full. This rule also applies to seeing a movie on an empty stomach – the multiplex is a nutritional disaster zone of popcorn, ice-cream and oversalted nuts. You may be the only person nibbling from a pack of trail mix, but so what? A small packet of unsalted nuts, fresh fruit, or a soy and linseed roll from the bakery make good portable snacks.

ONLY EAT WHEN YOU'RE HUNGRY

There's only one reason to eat and that's when you're actually hungry.

This may sound obvious until you start counting up the number of times you've eaten a biscuit, chocolate or cake, just because someone's offered it. Wait until your body, not the time or another person, tells you it's time to eat. That way you'll be more in tune with your body's cues that you're hungry.

Lean and green – the case for becoming vegetarian

The image of vegetarian eating is changing. For starters, the number of celebrities who've renounced eating meat has made a vegetarian diet look more hip than hippie. Concerns about the environment have also highlighted the fact that vegetarian, or semi-vegetarian, eating is kinder to the planet than the high meat consumption common to most industrialised countries. According to the Climate Institute, producing one kilo of beef results in more CO_2 emissions than going for a three-hour drive while leaving all the lights on at home.

A vegetarian diet can also keep you in better shape. One of the largest comparisons of the health of vegetarians with meat eaters, a UK study of 57,000 people in the late 1990s known as the Oxford Study, found that vegetarians had 25 per cent less heart disease and cancer, had lower blood pressure and were slimmer. More recently, researchers from the pro-vegetarian Physicians' Committee for Responsible Medicine in the US set out to see to how well a vegan diet worked for controlling diabetes compared with the eating guidelines from the American Diabetes Association. What they found was that the vegetarian option had a weight loss bonus. While people eating both diets improved their diabetes control, those on the vegetarian diet did best – *and* they lost weight, even though they had a kind of all-you-can-eat low fat vegan diet with no limits on carbs, kilojoules or portion sizes.

Then there's the 'Eco-Atkins' study from the father of the Glycaemic Index, Professor David Jenkins from the University of Toronto, who wondered what would happen if you swapped the protein from meat, eggs and cheese in an Atkins-style diet for protein from soy, nuts and gluten. After 28 weeks, a group of overweight men and women following a vegan diet had lost 10 per cent of their starting weight.

Skinnier waists weren't the only reward. Their insulin sensitivity had improved, lowering their risk of diabetes, and their cholesterol levels were better.

There are good reasons why vegetarian eating can help you lose weight and keep you healthier. Once you drop flesh foods from your diet, eating at least five serves of vegetables and two pieces of fruit a day is easy because there's more room for plant foods. With all those vegetables, fruits, nuts and legumes come a wide range of antioxidants and other healthy plant chemicals, along with a load of filling fibre that helps lower cholesterol and improve the health of your gut. And with less animal food comes less saturated fat. A pledge to veg also encourages you to experiment with lean nutritious foods like legumes and tofu, which you may not otherwise eat.

That said, it's also possible to eat a really unhealthy vegetarian diet – and even gain weight – if you eat the wrong foods. The most common mistakes people make when they try to go vegetarian are:

* *Not filling the nutrient gap left by taking animal foods off your plate.* It's not enough to eat meat and three veg minus the meat, or to eat pasta with a tomato sauce instead of a bolognaise sauce. You still need the protein, iron and zinc provided by meat or poultry. If you've sworn off dairy foods, then you're also missing out on calcium and vitamin B12.

* *Eating too many vegetarian foods that are high in 'bad' saturated fat.* What do chips, cake, pizza, vegetable pies, cheese and spinach quiche or deep fried vegetable samosas all have in common? They're all vegetarian . . . and all high in saturated fat and kilojoules. Lacto-ovo vegetarians (meaning vegetarians who include dairy food and eggs, as opposed to vegans who eat no animal foods at all) often use cheese as a major protein source – and this can be high in kilojoules and saturated fat.

How to make plant power work for you

Dairy products and eggs are both good sources of protein. Eating dairy products also makes it easier to get enough calcium as well as B12, a vitamin found mainly in meat, eggs and dairy products that is essential for avoiding a potentially serious type of anaemia. But you'll also need to eat plenty of legumes, nuts and seeds. These are all sources of plant protein, as well as iron and zinc.

If you decide to go vegan and ditch dairy and eggs, it becomes a little trickier. Without these foods, you need other ways of getting enough calcium (important for strong bones, especially after menopause) and enough B12. You need to eat enough plant foods containing calcium (calcium-fortified soy products like milk and yoghurt, almonds and dried figs are a few examples), and include foods fortified with B12 such as some soy milks and convenience vegetarian meals. Some yeast spreads, including Marmite, contain B12.

Plant protein – getting the balance right

While you can get protein from some plant foods like nuts, legumes and grains as well as meat, the type of protein differs. Meat, poultry, fish and other animal foods like dairy and eggs are what's called a 'complete protein' – they contain all the essential amino acids that work together like building blocks to make protein. Most plant protein foods, on the other hand, are an 'incomplete' protein – meaning they have *some* of the right amino acids, but not others. To get a complete protein you need to mix a number of plant foods together, e.g. combining a grain like rice or bread with legumes or nuts (think beans and rice, hummus and bread, or baked beans on toast). The advice used to be that you must eat the right mix of plant foods together at each meal. Now the rules have relaxed a bit and it's considered a good idea to eat a grain at one meal and legumes at the next.

Maxing your iron intake on a vegetarian diet

There's not just one kind of iron in food either. There's haem iron that is in animal foods, and non-haem iron in some plant foods and eggs. Your body absorbs haem iron from animals much better than non-haem iron from plants. You'll absorb more iron from plant foods, however, if you include vitamin C-rich vegetables – like tomatoes or red capsicum – at the same meal, or have a glass of orange juice. Say no to tea with meals – its tannins will block your absorption of iron from the legumes. But while female vegetarians can often be low in iron, there's some evidence that eating a vegetarian diet can also force the body to adjust to absorbing more non-haem iron from plant foods. Spinach, incidentally, does contain iron, but it's not the great iron source it's made out to be. It also contains something called oxalic acid that makes it hard for your body to absorb the iron. In other words, the iron is there, but you may not get as much – when it comes to greens, broccoli would give you a better iron boost than spinach .

Don't forget your zinc

Stirring yoghurt into a chickpea curry, or dunking wholegrain bread into yoghurt-based tzatziki dip could be a good move. According to research, adding yoghurt to a plant-based meal may help boost zinc absorption. This is worth knowing if you eat little or no meat, as a low intake of zinc, which is essential for a healthy immune system, is common among Australian women. Zinc levels may be especially low if you eat little or no red meat.

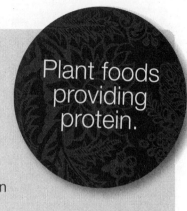

- 200 g cooked or canned beans, lentils or chickpeas = 15 g protein
- 200 g soy beans or soy products = 24 g protein
- 100 g tofu = 10 g protein
- 250 ml soy milk = 10 g protein
- 1 cup cooked brown rice = 6 g protein
- 1 cup cooked pasta = 6.8 g protein
- 50 g almonds = 10 g protein
- 1 cup sweet corn or 1 cup peas = 5 g protein
- 30 g seeds = 5 g protein

Plant foods providing protein.

With no studies directly comparing the health of people who eat only small amounts of meat, poultry or fish with that of more dedicated vegetarians, it's hard to know if you can still get all the benefits of a vegetarian diet. But eating less meat could help you lose weight – a study of more than 55,000 Swedish women who were middle-aged or older found that those who were vegetarian or semi-vegetarian and included fish in their diet tended to weigh less than meat eaters and were less likely to be overweight.

But for long-term good health, most nutrition experts agree that the best choice is a plant-based diet – meaning that most of the food that goes on your plate should come from plants, not animals. Studies show that the Mediterranean Diet (not the cream-based pasta dishes or tiramisu on offer at your local Italian eatery), which includes big helpings of vegetables, fruit, grains, legumes and nuts with some fish and olive oil, but only small amounts of meat or dairy products, has similar benefits to vegetarian diets, such as less heart disease and less risk of some cancers. It may even put the brakes on skin ageing: research at Melbourne's Monash University has linked a high intake of vegetables, fruit, olive oil and oily fish to fewer wrinkles, while full-fat milk, red meat and sugary foods appeared to increase skin damage.

While meat might still dominate the plates on many Australian tables, eating too much of it leaves less room for other important foods like fish and legumes, points out Accredited Practising Dietitian Monica Kubizniak of the Nutrition and Wellbeing Clinic in Sydney.

'You're getting protein, zinc and iron from meat, but you're not getting as much omega-3 fat as you would if you included more servings of fish,' she says.

'You're also missing out on the benefits of legumes such as beans, chickpeas and lentils, which can be the basis of meatless meals,' she adds.

There's no denying lean red meat can have real benefits for both health and weight loss. The downside is that fattier cuts are high in saturated fat, and a high intake of meat, especially processed meats like sausages and salami, has been increasingly linked to a higher risk of some cancers. In a study of 150,000 Americans, the American Cancer Society found that people eating the most processed meat – hot dogs, ham, bacon and salami – had twice the risk of bowel cancer compared with those who ate the least, while those who ate the most red meat had a 40 per cent higher risk. People who ate the most poultry or fish had a lower risk. The results of a study of more than half a million people across Europe, coordinated by the World Health Organization, found that those who ate 160 g or more of beef, lamb, veal or pork daily had a 35 per cent higher risk of bowel cancer – while eating 80 g of fish every day was linked to a 30 per cent lower risk.

As for what's behind the link between meat and cancer, that's not clear. Is there something in meat that contributes to cancer, or do larger servings of meat leave less room for the plant foods that may help prevent it? With processed meat, one suspect is thought to be the use of preservatives called nitrates and nitrites – the theory is that they can form cancer-causing substances in the gut. But with other meats, the problem may be how we cook it – cooking meat (and poultry and fish) at high temperatures, especially over open flames – can produce potentially carcinogenic chemicals called heterocyclic amines (HCAs), which can be absorbed when you eat, according to the American Institute for Cancer Research.

Other theories, suggests the Cancer Council of NSW, include meat's high iron content. While iron is essential, too much can cause free radical damage to the DNA of cells, making them vulnerable to cancer. Meat's fat content may also boost production of bile acid which can fuel cell growth in the lining of the colon – a problem if there are any malignant cells around. Omega-3 fatty acids in fish, on the other hand, seem to do the opposite and reduce cell growth. Another possible theory is that when undigested protein from meat arrives in your colon, it's eaten up by bacteria that then produce ammonia, which is a potential carcinogen. This is where a big salad or stir-fried vegetables with starchy food like rice or noodles come to the rescue. They encourage the growth of other bacteria that help mop up the ammonia.

Because it's important to get enough protein, iron and zinc if you're eating less meat, remember to eat some legumes or nuts. Eat legume-based dishes two or three times a week if you're eating some flesh foods – but have them daily if you choose to eat no meat, poultry or fish at all.

Plant foods and menopause

Can lean plant foods help with menopause symptoms too? I wish I could say yes, but although there's been some research suggesting that foods containing weak plant hormones called phytoestrogens (phyto means plant) can be helpful, the evidence isn't strong. The theory is that these plant versions of our own hormones – found in soy and other legumes like chickpeas, lentils and beans, as well as grains – help reduce some menopausal symptoms when our own ovaries start producing less oestrogen.

I was about 40 when I began reading some of the early studies into this – along with other research suggesting that fitter women often have an easier run through menopause too. I decided I'd be my own experiment – get as fit as possible and learn to cook with more soy foods and other legumes. For me, menopause arrived bang on schedule at 51, the average age. But I don't know what a hot flush feels like because I never had one. Nor did I have any other symptoms like night sweats or mood swings that some women report. The only difference to my life was I stopped buying tampons. I'm not saying it was the chickpeas and exercise that gave me a dream run (20 per cent of women have no symptoms at menopause and maybe I'm one of them) but it's worth thinking about, especially given that these high-fibre foods have other health benefits – soy, for instance, can help lower cholesterol.

But according to Sandra Villella, a naturopath with the Jean Hailes Foundation for Women's Health, women do vary in the way their bodies metabolise phytoestrogens, so not all women get a benefit from them. But if you want to give it a go, she suggests aiming for 200 g of tofu or tempeh or two cups of soybeans daily. These amounts are suggested to get the 40–80 mg of isoflavones (weak plant oestrogens) recommended to achieve a therapeutic effect, she says. These foods are also a better bet than more processed soy foods like soy milk, soy yoghurt and soy-based meat replacements.

Breads that include soy flour are good to include too, as are other legumes like chickpeas, lentils and beans. They also contain plant hormones, but not as much as soy. She suggests, however, that women with an underactive thyroid should avoid soy. She also recommends giving soy supplements a miss, especially if you have a personal or family history of breast cancer.

Before you buy a weight loss supplement, read this

If there is a dieter's Holy Grail, it's the idea that putting something into your mouth, as opposed to *not* putting something into your mouth, can help the kilos drop off. Browse the shelves of pharmacies, health food stores and supermarkets and, with so many products claiming to suppress appetite and boost metabolism, dropping a dress size should be a breeze.

But despite their use of big words like 'thermogenic' or 'fat metaboliser', which imply they have scientific cred, there's little solid research to match many of their claims. The story so far is that there's *some* evidence to suggest *some* ingredients in weight loss products, including green tea, bitter orange and capsaicin (the active ingredient that gives chilli its bite), can increase metabolism *a little*, but this doesn't necessarily translate into weight loss. The effect on metabolism is small, the evidence isn't strong and more studies are needed, says nutritionist Dr Rosemary Stanton. Caffeine and guarana (a plant extract containing caffeine), other common ingredients in weight loss products, can also boost metabolism slightly, she says – but again the effect is small and only lasts for a couple of weeks.

Almost ten years ago Dr Stanton and other experts wrote a review published in the *Medical Journal of Australia* looking at what scientific research says about the effectiveness of common ingredients in non-prescription weight loss supplements The ingredients studied included brindleberry, chitosan, capsaicin, caffeine, L-carnitine, chromium picolinate, gingko biloba, a seaweed called fucus vesiculosus, fibre supplements, grapeseed extract, lecithin, St John's wort, isoflavones and horse chestnut. The review concluded that there was little evidence to support the use of any of them. Since then, not much has changed in the way of stronger evidence or promising new supplements, says Rosemary.

An appetite suppressant made from an African plant called *hoodia gordonii* is one of few new developments. Traditionally used by Kalahari bushmen to suppress appetite and thirst on hunting trips, it appears to work on the part of the brain that tells you when you've eaten enough. Some animal studies and one human study found that taking hoodia reduced kilojoule intake, and at the time of writing, there are studies going ahead in Europe to find out more. As for hoodia supplements touted on the internet, there's no guarantee that they're even the real thing, let alone that they actually work.

The problem for consumers is that many claims for weight loss supplements don't reflect the often flimsy or non-existent evidence that the ingredients work, even though price tags can be as high as $60. When I interviewed Rosemary Stanton for *The Sydney Morning Herald*, I asked her to look at the information provided for a product promoted as 'the first weight loss and weight control formula for peri- menopausal and post-menopausal women'.

'Hormonal and metabolic changes around menopause make it harder for women to maintain their ideal weight and body shape', read the hype, but the supplement, it said, would help boost metabolic rate to help burn fat faster. By 'balancing hormones and blood sugar levels', it would help protect against weight gain and altering body shape during hormone changes.

This might sound like music to the ears of women struggling with weight gain, but it sounded like rubbish to Rosemary Stanton. There's no evidence that hormonal changes at menopause cause weight gain, she says, and no evidence that the ingredients in this product, such as iodine, chromium, vitex or chasteberry, help with weight loss.

It might be news to you that, unlike prescription and non-prescription drugs, which must meet requirements for safety, quality and efficacy, complementary medicines, including weight loss supplements, aren't evaluated to see if they actually work by the Therapeutic Goods Administration, the office of the Department of Health and Ageing that regulates medicines in Australia.

So before you hand over your money for a product:

* Ask the pharmacist what the evidence is to support the claims.
* Think about what the product information on the pack really says. Typical phrases such as 'may assist in weight loss' are not exactly a money-back guarantee that it works. The packaging may also say an ingredient has been 'traditionally' used for weight loss. 'Traditional use' doesn't mean it works or that there's

evidence to back it up. Claims that a product 'provides weight loss support', 'helps fatigue brought about by diet and exercise', or 'assists with imbalances' are not the same as saying it will actually help you lose weight.

* The product is likely to say it should be used in conjunction with a healthy eating and exercise plan. In other words, better habits, not pills, are still the best way to lose weight.

Action list

- Include both lean protein and a healthy carb at each meal.

- Don't let yourself get too hungry. Carry healthy snacks (fruit or nuts) with you if you're going somewhere with no access to healthy food.

- Don't overload your plate (you're likely to eat it, hungry or not). Start with a smaller serving and add more if you're still hungry.

- Invest your money in fresh, healthy food – not weight loss supplements.

Chapter 6

Planning for a healthier waist

*D*id you know that fat on different parts of you behaves in different ways? The fat on female thighs and buttocks can be healthy, producing friendly chemicals that can prevent diabetes by helping insulin work better. Excess weight around the middle, on the other hand, is a clue that you're carrying a troublesome type of fat called visceral fat. This is why being pear-shaped and overweight is healthier than being an overweight 'apple' – the kind of body shape where weight is concentrated around the middle.

So what's so bad about visceral fat? Unlike the fat that you can pinch just under your skin (called subcutaneous fat), visceral fat lies below the muscles and does more than just sit there doing nothing much. Many researchers now see this kind of fat with new eyes – not just as something that sits and makes muffin tops, but that acts like an organ in its own right, producing inflammatory chemicals that can cause mischief, such as damaging arteries and increasing diabetes risk. It also spills out fatty acids that can make the liver produce more cholesterol.

These inflammatory chemicals are meant to be friendly. They're part of the immune system and their job description is to repair damaged tissue and help destroy organisms that cause infection. When a splinter hurts your finger or bacteria invade your throat, for instance, your immune system sends out a cavalry of inflammatory chemicals to help you heal. The inflammation that follows is caused by extra blood flow to the injured or infected area, and is all part of the repair process that makes things better. But sometimes the immune system misfires – an allergic reaction like asthma, for instance, is a result of a trigger-happy immune system that overreacts. It's a similar story with these inflammatory chemicals. Scientists think that some people have a chronic inflammation hidden in the body that doesn't turn off.

It's now thought that it's not 'bad' LDL cholesterol working alone that gums up arteries, causing heart attack and stroke, but a combination of both inflammation and cholesterol. Inflammation can also be the final straw that triggers a heart attack – it can cause an already bulging artery wall to crack open, creating a blockage. Chronic inflammation interferes with the function of insulin to other parts of the body, making it harder to keep blood sugar levels normal. It may also increase the risk of Alzheimer's disease as well.

Should I get liposuction to shift the fat?

Sorry, it's not much help here – while it can get rid of the subcutaneous fat that lies under the surface of your skin, it can't get rid of deeper visceral fat around your organs – this means that liposuction doesn't reduce your risk of health problems related to being overweight, such as heart disease and diabetes. Researchers in the US studying the effects of liposuction on women with insulin resistance – the condition that can lead to diabetes – found that 12 weeks after the procedure there was no significant improvement in their insulin resistance or in their levels of blood fats. Not only that, but liposuction is really only a very temporary solution to weight loss unless you're prepared to exercise more and eat a healthier diet, points out Dr Anand Ramakrishnan, a spokesperson for the Australian Society of Plastic Surgeons.

'To a degree, liposuction improves appearance in a cosmetic sense, but as you get older, new fat cells are formed and if you don't change your lifestyle,' he explains, 'these cells will fill up with more fat.'

So if there's enough money in the bank to pay for liposuction, use it to join a gym or hire a personal trainer to help you make real changes that will benefit your health as well as your body shape.

Can sit-ups help?

No, no and *no*. Done correctly, crunches and other abdominal exercise will strengthen abdominal muscles – but they can't get rid of the layer of fat on top of them. You'll just end up with strong muscles hidden under a potbelly.

Heart disease? Who, me?

If you're like most women, you probably spend more time worrying about the health of your partner's arteries than your own – men, after all, generally have a higher risk of heart disease than women. But by the time women reach menopause, the risk factors start piling up and women and men have the same probability of having a heart attack at midlife.

Higher levels of oestrogen are the reason why a woman's risk of heart disease before menopause is lower than a man's. But when levels drop, her risk of heart disease goes up. And while breast cancer might be the disease women worry about most, it's not the one that's most likely to be the death of them – heart disease kills around four times as many women as breast cancer.

Weight gain around the waist boosts your risk of other problems that increase your chances of heart disease, such as increased blood pressure, high cholesterol levels and insulin resistance.

How to be a proactive eater

Proactive eating means thinking ahead and planning what you'll eat. It's usually smarter than being a reactive eater, who operates without a plan and reacts to hunger by eating whatever's within easy reach, regardless of its nutritional quality.

Eating healthier and skinnier is as much about planning as it is about nutrition. The same excuse offered up for not exercising, 'I don't have time', is also a reason for relying on convenience food that makes it hard

It took about three years for library assistant Sally Turansky to grow two dress sizes – a journey she blames partly on snacking between meals. Now, having dumped the dips, chips and cheese – and the size 14s – she's wearing a size 10. The crunch came when Sally, 53, realised she couldn't zip up her pants, while her partner was told by his doctor that he needed to shed weight around the waist too. And 16 months after switching to a healthier way of eating – fruit between meals, big helpings of vegetables at lunch and dinner – and more exercise – they've both lost weight. Sally's 'bad' LDL cholesterol has dropped and the roll of fat around her waist has disappeared.

'There's no point in going on a diet – you have to change your way of eating permanently and exercise more,' says Sally, who now fits in four hours of walking each week, including some hills, along with a weekly game of tennis and sessions on the rowing machine at home. On weekends away and holidays, she paddles her kayak for up to two hours, which she considers a workout for her mind as well as her body.

'We feel so much better,' she says, 'and we've thrown out all our fat clothes!'

to keep to a healthier weight. This is especially true of that most squeezed of meals: weeknight dinners when you may be tired, hungry or stressed and need food fast.

But would you start the working week with no plan to tackle the Monday to Friday workload? Healthy eating is no different. You should use the same organised approach to the week's eating as you would to your job.

If there's healthy food in the house that's quick to cook, then that's what you'll eat. Stocking the fridge and pantry with the right stuff means you can:

* **Feed yourself lean, nutrient-dense food** so you're less likely to need extra snacks.

* *Make healthy dinners fast*. These are the meals that are a result of forward planning – you look at the week ahead and get a rough idea of what to eat.
* *Produce 'panic' food* at times when you need healthy food in a hurry – you're home late, there's no time/energy to cook, or you're going out and need a mini-meal beforehand – situations when you might normally rely on fast food.

Learn to fast-track midweek dinners

Decide what to eat for the week ahead and work out what cooking/meal preparation you can do in advance to take the pressure off the busiest weeknights. This buys more time to do active stuff in the evenings, such as a yoga class or going for a walk.

Spending a couple of hours cooking, or partially cooking, two or three dishes at weekends makes a difference – if you're dicing onions for one dish you may as well dice for two. The best cook-ahead dishes are those you can reheat quickly, or those that need no reheating, like curries, casseroles, a pesto sauce for pasta, or roast vegetables to toss with leafy greens for weeknight salads or for brown-bagging lunches for work. Suggestions include:

SOUP

Make it with legumes and it's substantial enough for a mid-week meal rounded out with a big salad and some sourdough or pita bread with hummus or baba ganoush. It can also be left to simmer on the stove while you prepare the rest of your meal.

STEAMED BASMATI, BROWN RICE, COUS COUS OR KAMUT

provides the base for a one-pot meal of fried rice with lots of vegetables and nuts, like cashews or pistachios. Or have cooked rice ready to heat up with a stir-fry, or the foundation of a grain-based salad to take to work.

ROAST VEGETABLES

A batch of carrots and sweet potato (cut into chunks), red onions (quartered), sprayed with a little oil, can roast in a hot oven (around 45 minutes) while you're making a soup or a curry. Whole beetroot is good too (but add more cooking time depending on size). Add some crushed garlic, herbs and black pepper or dukkah for extra flavour. Roast vegetables like this add variety and substance to mid-week salads. Good combinations include sweet potato and baby spinach leaves, or roast beetroot with rocket, fresh mint and a little crumbled fetta or goat's cheese. You can also bake a few capsicums whole until the skins blacken and blister. Putting them in a plastic bag until they cool makes it easy to peel off the skin, ready for adding to salads.

Does your kitchen need a makeover?

Audit the contents of your cupboard, fridge and freezer, and boot out anything that:

* offers little in the way of nutrition. Why buy something that's all kilojoules with no decent nutrients, such as snack foods, fizzy drinks, sweets and biscuits?
* is high in unhealthy fats (saturated fat or trans fats), e.g. croissants, commercial cakes, frozen pizza and creamy dips
* is based on unsmart carbs, e.g. lightweight breakfast cereals, cakes and biscuits (again), cake mixes and white bread
* is highly processed, especially meats such as ham, bacon and salami.

In the cupboard – what stays in?

* *Olive oil* and *olive oil spray*.
* *Sesame oil*, to add flavour to stir fries.
* *Peanut oil*, for stir-fries. It has a higher smoke point so it's better for stir-frying.
* *Canned fish* for quick salads and pastas, or to add protein (and omega-3 fats) to risotto and stir-fries. Don't overlook sardines packed in spring water (an inexpensive source of omega-3). Mash with lemon juice or vinegar and eat on toasted sourdough.
* *Anchovies*. Just a few anchovies mashed into canned tomatoes with a few capers, olives, crushed garlic and chilli make a fast pasta sauce.
* *Canned legumes* like cannelini beans, chickpeas, red kidney beans and black beans (see Legumes 101 on page 135).
* *Dried red and green lentils*.
* *Canned tomatoes*.
* Cans of *corn kernels*, which are good with brown rice salads or combined with black beans.
* Jars of *baby beetroot*. Drain and toss with vinaigrette for a fast side dish – add fresh herbs (mint and dill are great), sumac or cumin with freshly ground black pepper.
* A good *pasta sauce*.
* *Seeded mustard* – for making salad dressings, or to use as a spread with sandwiches and wraps.
* *Pasta*.
* *Basmati rice*.
* *Brown rice*.
* *Arborio rice* for risotto.
* *Bulghur*. Fine bulghur (cracked wheat) is good in tabouleh salad, but you can also buy coarse bulghur for making grain-based dishes.
* *Quinoa*.
* *Barley*.

- *Bread*. Choose dense, wholegrain breads, rye pita bread, oat or rye mountain bread, sourdough bread or pumpernickel.
- *Wholemeal tortillas* are good for wraps and beany burritos.
- *Rolled oats*.
- *Dried fruit*.
- *Nuts and seeds* (though it's better to keep them in the fridge – they stay fresher longer). Apart from their snack value, a supply of cashews, walnuts and pine nuts means you've always got an easy source of protein to add to a quick stir-fry, vegetarian curry or a salad.
- *Muesli* – preferably the one you made yourself.
- *Lemon and lime juice*.
- *Asian sauces* (but use sparingly – they're high in sodium).
- *Good curry paste*.

Herbs and spices.

Everyone has their own favourites – the following are really versatile:

Turmeric: The yellow spice, rich in an antioxidant called curcumin, has been linked to a lower risk of some cancers and Alzheimer's disease. Adding black pepper may help your body absorb more curcumin. It's good for use in curries, Middle Eastern dishes and added to rice.

Cumin: Cumin teams really well with legumes like chickpeas, black beans and red kidney beans.

Sumac: This is a dark red Middle Eastern spice, which is good in sauces and works well with rice, cous cous or bulgur. Alternatively, sprinkle on salads or roast vegetables.

Dukkah: Dukkah is more substantial than a spice because it's a blend of toasted nuts, seeds and spices. Sprinkle on salads or yoghurt dips or stir into vegetable dishes.

Zatar: This is another Middle Eastern blend of herbs and spices, often with mint, thyme and sumac. Try it in salads, rice dishes or with poultry.

In the fridge

* *Healthy, plant-based dips.* Use them as spreads on bread, or with raw vegetables as a snack, e.g. baba ganoush or tzatziki. Check the labels and choose those lowest in saturated fat. Dips containing cheese are likely to be higher in saturated fat. Most dips freeze well. A couple of different dips in the fridge can also help wean you off a heavy cheese habit – dips made with pulses (e.g. hummus) or with nuts contain some protein and make a change from cheese in wraps and sandwiches.

* *Margarine and butter.* It's up to you, but I think there are healthier things to spread on bread and toast – low fat ricotta, a little olive oil, the dips mentioned above, or mashed avocado with black pepper. These foods add nutrients and healthier types of fat. Butter is high in saturated fat, but remember that eating too many vegetable oils from the omega-6 family on which many margarines are based – think safflower and corn oil (see Chapter 5) – isn't a great idea either. They're one of the reasons for the imbalance of fatty acids in a typical Western diet. However, if your cholesterol level needs to come down, there's evidence that spreads containing plant sterols can help.

* *Parmesan, fetta cheese and goat's cheese.* These cheeses have strong flavours so a little goes a long way. .

* *Firm tofu.* For stir-fries.

* *Organic or free-range eggs.* Avoid cage eggs. Organic usually taste the best.

* *Salad leaves.* If you buy them ready bagged, look for the pack with the longest shelf life.

Fresh vegetables and fruit

* *Fresh herbs*. Apart from their health benefits, fresh herbs can make even really basic food special. Try fresh mint, coriander or Thai basil in a stir-fry, basil or oregano on tomatoes and mushrooms on toast or in salads, parsley in scrambled eggs, rosemary with roast vegetables. Never be stingy with fresh herbs – especially parsley, mint and basil. Mint keeps well and is really versatile – wonderful in salads, stir-fries and teamed with yoghurt-based dips and sauces. Extend the lifespan of herbs by storing them washed and wrapped in kitchen paper in a plastic container in the fridge. The exception is basil, which should be sealed in a plastic bag to avoid any exposure to the chilly air in the fridge – this will turn it black fast. If you want a good standby, supermarkets sell herbs in tubes in the fruit and veg section.
* *Fresh chilli*. Even if you're no fan of fiery food, just a sliver or two can be enough to lift the flavour of food without making it hot. If you don't use a lot, keep a few in a container in the freezer.
* *Root ginger*. Use generously in stir-fries. It can also be frozen.

In the freezer

* Foods that will keep well in the freezer for two or three months include smoked salmon, wholegrain or sourdough bread; small lean portions of fish, poultry and meat if you eat them; pizza bases, fresh rice noodles; frozen vegetables; frozen berries; nuts and seeds if you buy them in bulk .

Savvier supermarket shopping

When you're on a mission to do food shopping fast, it's so easy to pluck something off the shelf because the big print on the front of the package makes it sound healthy or skinny. Organic, 98 per cent fat free, high in fibre, fortified with folate and iron, cholesterol free, natural or even vegetarian all seem to be other ways of saying foods are healthy. But are they really?

Sometimes. But while a packet of breakfast cereal can trumpet virtues like low in fat, high in vitamins and minerals on the front of the pack, reading the teensy weensy print on the nutrition panel can tell you a different story – that it's high in sugar or low in fibre. Ditto yoghurt – sometimes there's not much difference in kilojoules between low fat, no fat yoghurt and the full fat versions, because the manufacturers have added extra sugar and carbohydrates to the supposedly skinnier yoghurt to make up for less fat. When a food wears a low fat/fat free label it's not a licence to eat as much as you like. Organic? Reducing the pesticide load on us and the environment is a good move – but before you decide it's an impeccable choice, check the nutrition panel and ask if the product ticks other boxes too. Is it low in saturated fat, sugar and sodium?

It's also smart to avoid processed food where possible, and head for the foods that aren't plastered with confusing information, namely fresh fruit and vegetables.

Read what the label really says

NO CHOLESTEROL

This doesn't necessarily mean a food is healthy or even that it's low in fat or kilojoules – oils don't contain cholesterol, for instance. The main thing to remember is that what causes high levels of cholesterol is eating too much of the wrong kind of fats – it's this that encourages your body to make too much cholesterol. Cholesterol is produced in your liver and, when you eat too much saturated fat (or trans fats), your liver produces too much cholesterol.

NATURAL

The word 'natural' is meaningless – it doesn't mean a food is healthier. As for light or lite – this can mean the colour is light, as in light olive oil, so it's no guarantee of fewer kilojoules.

TRANS FATS

Trans fatty acids (TFAs) are created when food processing hydrogenates (hardens) vegetable fats to make them firmer, and they are even more harmful than saturated fat. Like saturated fat, trans fats raise bad LDL cholesterol but they also lower good HDL cholesterol, which is bad news if you're approaching menopause and the increased risk of heart disease that goes with it. And if that's not bad enough, new research from France has also linked high levels of trans fats in the diet to an increased risk of breast cancer.

Although small amounts of trans fats occur naturally in meat and dairy products, most trans fats in our food got there via food processing. To avoid it, check the labels on margarine for their TFA content, and steer clear of processed foods, especially cakes and biscuits, and fast food. Ingredients such as 'hydrogenated vegetable oil' or 'partially hydrogenated vegetable oil' on food labels are clues that the product contains TFAs.

There's also evidence that trans fatty acids may be inflammatory too. Researchers at Harvard Medical School have reported that women who ate the most trans fatty acids also had the highest levels of inflammatory markers in their blood.

SALT

Salt in food won't add kilos, but its sodium content can raise blood pressure. By making your body retain extra fluid, excess salt can increase the volume of blood flowing through your arteries. This makes your heart work harder, increasing blood pressure, along with the risk of heart disease and stroke. Excess salt can also 'age' your arteries by making them stiff and old before their time.

In Australia, the advice is to keep salt intake to less than 6 g of salt (or about 2300 mg of sodium) daily, which is a little more than one teaspoon of salt a day. Yet, on average, we eat about 9 g a day, mainly because we're not the only ones holding the salt shaker. About 75 per cent of our sodium intake comes from salt added by the food industry. Around 15 per cent is what we add ourselves.

The remaining 10 per cent comes from sodium that's naturally in food – an amount that supplies all we need. But even if you give most processed food a wide berth, it's hard to keep excess salt out of your diet. Just five slices of bread can provide as much as 1150 mg of sodium, which is half the daily upper limit, while one tablespoon of soy sauce in a stir-fry can add 1000 mg of sodium.

It's best to keep processed food to a minimum and become familiar with the difference between low salt food (one with less than 120 mg of sodium per 100 g) and high salt food (one with 600 mg of sodium per 100 g). It's also worth comparing the salt content of different breads, as some are higher than others.

As for avoiding extra salt when you cook, some natural flavours are better at pumping up flavour than others. Try chilli, garlic, fresh ginger, fresh herbs, lime and lemon juice and dried mushrooms. When you're making Asian food, adding extra garlic, ginger, chilli and mint or Thai basil means you need less fish or soy sauce. If you do use salt, iodised salt is best.

Ingredient	A little (grams per 100 g)	A lot (grams per 100 g)
Sugar	5 g	15 g
Saturated fat	1 g	5 g
Dietary fibre	0.5 g	3 g
Sodium (salt)	0.1 g	0.5 g

Nutrition panels – what to look for.

Why you need more plants on your plate

Not long ago I joined some neighbours for a barbecue, but what was different about this one is that the vegetables were the star turn. On a long table in the garden, there was a vast bowl of salad niçoise, glistening with olives and ripe tomatoes; another roast vegetable salad, a dish of baked onion and potato, a whole fish baked with more vegetables and, finally, at the end of the table, almost like an afterthought, a plate of meat from the barbecue. Maybe it was because this particular neighbour comes from Southern France where salad and raw vegetables are taken more seriously, but the point of this story is that we need to make a similar shift in our attitude to food – focus more on vegetables and eat smaller amounts of meat.

Eating more vegetables, fruit, legumes, wholegrains and nuts gets more important than ever at midlife. They help keep you leaner, provide plant chemicals that may help prevent cancer, and they protect your heart in three different ways – with artery-friendly antioxidants, plant fibres (in soy, barley, oats and nuts) that keep bad LDL cholesterol down and with potassium to keep blood pressure down.

Don't believe anyone who tells you it's normal for blood pressure to rise with age. It's not. High blood pressure, which increases the risk of heart disease and stroke, is the planet's third leading cause of death and disability.

In the past, studies of traditional societies that didn't depend on processed food, found that high blood pressure was almost unknown. It's partly because, thanks to a diet of natural food, they ate much more potassium than sodium, which is just the way it's meant to be. But a typical Western diet, high in processed food, gives us the reverse: levels of sodium that are higher than potassium.

So while we need to reduce sodium by eating less salt, less processed food and going easy on the fish sauce, we also need more vegetables and fruit to pump up the potassium in our diets. When wholegrains are refined to create lightweight bread and breakfast cereal, out goes the potassium, along with the fibre.

While it's not hard to eat enough fruit, a minimum of five serves of vegetables each day can be challenging for some people, especially if they wait until dinner to fit them all in.

Five serves minimum a day

Five serves of vegetables isn't a huge amount – one serve = half a cup of cooked vegetable or one cup of salad.

For a reality check of how much veg you're eating (or not eating), keep a food diary for a week to see how many serves you're getting and where you might be missing out. The next step is to find ways to include vegetables in meals and snacks throughout the day rather than leaving it all until dinner. Add two or three salad vegetables to a sandwich at lunch, or eat a salad.

You could also:

* snack on a slice of soy and linseed or sourdough toast with chopped ripe tomatoes or mashed avocado on top
* add two or three extra vegetables to curries or pasta sauces
* make extra salad or vegetables for dinner and take for lunch the next day.
* eat greens with everything – add leafy veg like spinach, rocket and pak choy to risottos, soups and pasta sauces, or curries and pilafs – just stir them in towards the end of cooking and let them wilt.
* buy bagged salads or pre-chopped stir-fried vegetables to save time (look for the packs with the longest shelf life)
* toss slices of oiled eggplant, zucchini and capsicum onto the barbecue.

Add vegetables to weekend breakfasts

With more time to eat, weekends are an opportunity to pack in an extra serve or two of vegetables – cooking in a little olive oil adds extra flavour and helps you absorb more antioxidants from the vegetables. You could:

* make a vegetable frittata
* cook ripe tomatoes with garlic and basil and serve with eggs or baked beans on wholegrain toast
* cook tomatoes, garlic and mushrooms on toasted sourdough bread
* stir-fry spinach with pine nuts and garlic and pile on wholegrain toast spread with low fat ricotta
* cook tomatoes, onions, garlic and capsicum in olive oil until soft and mushy. Pour into a shallow ovenproof dish. For four people, make four wells in the vegetable mixture. Crack four free range eggs and pour one into each well. Bake in a moderate oven until the eggs are poached – 15 to 20 minutes.

How to make salads with substance

Learning to make a range of different salads with different flavours and textures solves a lot of problems. What can I eat without messing up saucepans? How can I get more fibre and how can I fill half my plate with vegetables I really want to eat? If you make a big enough salad for dinner, you'll have lunch to take to work the next day.

Salads aren't just about leaves – just about any plant food can work as a salad ingredient (even stale bread), so don't be afraid to experiment with different grains, nuts and legumes as well as vegetables. Steaming some vegetables (really lightly so they stay crisp) adds different textures. Broccoli and carrot are examples of vegetables which deliver more of some of their nutrients when they're lightly steamed as opposed to eaten raw, because the cooking process can release more of the phytochemicals from the plant cells.

You can put salad on the table as an extra dish at most evening meals (the only time the salad bowl is missing from my table is when we're eating stir-fried vegetables). It's a simple way to add another serve or two of vegetables and acts as extra filler. If you chomp your way through enough veg at dinner, you're less likely to be snacking in front of the TV later on.

Follow these rules to upgrade your salad bowl:

- *Lose the iceberg* in favour of darker, more nutrient-dense leaves like cos, spinach, rocket, radicchio, mizuna or tatsoi. They're high in folate – credited with helping prevent heart disease. Dark green leaves are also an easy way to scoop up eye-friendly nutrients lutein and zeaxanthin, which may help protect against age-related macular degeneration.

- *Don't stop at two or three ingredients.* The more you add, the wider the variety of nutrients you'll capture in one bowl and the more interesting the salad. Think ripe red or yellow tomatoes, radish, raw or roasted red onion, avocado, red or orange capsicum, red cabbage, snow peas, broccoli, slices of steamed baby potatoes, fresh basil or mint.

- *Forget the no-fat dressing.* Remember, a little good fat like olive oil in a dressing helps you absorb more antioxidants from the veg.

- *Add protein to turn your salad into a main meal* with lean, skinless chicken, chunks of canned tuna, hard boiled eggs, pine nuts or chickpeas.

- *Add texture.* Firmer ingredients like roasted sweet potato, very lightly steamed cauliflower or asparagus, cannellini beans, fresh peas, nuts or toasted seeds give extra body and bulk.

- *Use grains as a salad base.* For more filling power, base salads on cooked grains like brown or basmati rice, noodles, cous cous or bulgur (soaked or cooked) – be sure they're completely cool before mixing with raw vegetables.

- *Keep a range of salad add-ons* in the fridge or on the shelf to add flavour and interest – capers, anchovies, pine nuts, walnuts, artichoke hearts, olives, parmesan and reduced-fat fetta. The spice blend, dukkah, is great sprinkled on either a grain-based or a leafy salad.

- *Add salad sprouts.* Sprouted beans like mung beans, lentils or chickpeas have good things going for them – besides boosting their nutrient content, the sprouting process also makes them less wind-producing than unsprouted beans. The megastars of the sprout world are broccoli sprouts – researchers at Johns Hopkins University in the US have estimated that three-day-old broccoli sprouts contain 20 to 50 times the cancer fighting compounds as mature broccoli (great news for non-lovers of broccoli). Compared to the vegetable itself, sprouts have a much milder taste.

* *Add dressing to leafy salads just before serving*, otherwise the leaves will turn soggy. Don't overdress a salad – it's best to start off with a small amount and add more if you need it.

DIY salad dressing

Why bother with commercial salad dressing? In the time it takes to track it down in the supermarket, you can whip it up at home and know exactly what's in it. Most bought dressings are heavy on sodium. If you make your own, you've got more control of the ingredients. Olive oil, especially virgin olive oil, contains a naturally occurring anti-inflammatory called oleocanthol which may help reduce the risk of heart disease and dementia. As for vinegar, when it's eaten with other food, it may help lower blood sugar by slowing the rate at which carbohydrates are digested. And garlic can help lower blood pressure, as well as bad LDL cholesterol.

Simple vinaigrette

As a rough guide, use half extra virgin olive with half white balsamic vinegar and add your own favourite flavours – crushed garlic, a Dijon-style mustard, a little honey, chilli or lemon zest.

¼ cup olive oil

¼ cup white balsamic vinegar (not dark balsamic which can overpower the flavour of salad veg)

1 clove of garlic, crushed

1 teaspoon Dijon-style mustard

1 teaspoon honey

squeeze of lemon juice

grated rind of half a lemon

a pinch of chilli flakes

Even better vinaigrettes:

Roast garlic vinaigrette

For a really thick, garlicky dressing, shave a thin slice off the top of a whole bulb of garlic, spray with oil, wrap in foil and bake in a hot oven (about 15 minutes) until the cloves soften and ooze out of their skin. Buzz the garlic with the vinaigrette in a blender/food processor. This is a great dressing for potato salad instead of mayo.

Roast capsicum vinaigrette

Take two even-sized capsicums and slice off the stalk end to form a lid. Stand the capsicums in a baking tray, fill the cavities with vinaigrette, replace the lid and enclose the capsicum in foil. Bake in a hot oven for about 45 minutes. Take the capsicum out of the oven, empty the dressing (now flavoured with roast capsicum) and store in a bottle. Seal the cooked capsicums in a plastic bag until cool (this makes them easier to peel, although they're okay unpeeled too). Add the dressing and roast capsicum to a salad of leaves and pine nuts.

Asian salad dressing

¼ cup olive oil

1 tablespoon fish sauce

2 tablespoons lime juice

½ to 1 tablespoons soy sauce

crushed garlic

A little chopped fresh chilli

1–2 teaspoons palm sugar or raw sugar

1 teaspoon grated ginger

This is good added to a mix of shredded Chinese cabbage, shredded carrot, shallots, cucumber, fresh mint and coriander or Thai basil. You can toss in some chopped nuts and cooked, cooled noodles for more substance.

'But vegetables go off so quickly'

This is a common reason for missing out on vegetables. Solve it by:

- buying vegetables as *fresh* as possible
- choosing vegetables with a *longer fridge life*. E.g. Cos lettuce, capsicum, carrots, Chinese cabbage (wombok), red cabbage, sweet corn, radish. Sweet potato is good too, but store it out of the fridge in a cool, dark place
- have some *frozen* vegetables as back-up
- buy *unripened* avocadoes
- *use* more perishable vegetables, like salad leaves, first.

Why it's good to mix up your grains

Pasta, bread, cracked wheat and cous cous might be different, but they're all from a single grain – wheat. But replacing some wheat with other wholegrains like oats, barley, rice or rye gives you a broader mix of nutrients, including heart-healthy fibres and plant hormones that are good to include at midlife. These grains are also low, or lower, GI.

Grain benefits.

Traditional or steel cut oats. Compared to quick cooking or instant oats, these less refined oats are slowly absorbed, helping you feel full long after eating breakfast. They also deliver nutrients – B vitamins, vitamin E, protein and minerals, as well as a fibre called beta-glucan, which helps sweep cholesterol out of the body.

Cooking traditional oats doesn't take long – use about one part rolled oats to four parts water (or water and milk, preferably low fat). Speed up cooking by pouring hot water over them the instant you get out of bed. Let them stand while you shower. If you're using steel cut oats, soak them the night before.

BARLEY

Nutty, filling and rich in heart-healthy beta-glucan, you can add barley to slow-cooking soups and casseroles. It makes a good nutty-flavoured risotto, especially teamed with wilted greens and parmesan – but be prepared to stay longer at the stove. There are two kinds of barley – unrefined barley (usually just labelled 'barley') and pearl barley. Although pearl barley has had its husk removed, it's still good because its fibre is distributed throughout the grain, not just on the outside.

RYE

Containing plant oestrogens called lignans, rye may help lower the risk of heart disease. Many rye breads are a mix of rye and wheat. Darker rye breads usually contain more rye. Pumpernickel is 100 per cent rye. You can also add rolled rye to muesli.

BROWN RICE

This wonder grain has three times the fibre of white rice and, at 350 kJ (or 85 calories) for half a cup, has a place on any weight loss plan. Because it's gluten free and relatively non-allergenic, it's good for anyone with a food intolerance or allergies. Compared to white rice, brown rice has more vitamin E and more protein. Mixed with beans and chopped vegetables, it makes a filling and portable salad to take to work. It's good for fried rice too. Brown rice is another slow cooker – steam plenty at once and freeze in batches to use later.

QUINOA (PRONOUNCED KEEN-WAH)

A fast cooking, high protein South American food that cooks like a grain, Quinoa is really the seed of a grass. Like cous cous, it combines well with strong flavoured ingredients.

Quinoa is great mixed with onion, capsicum, roast sweet potato and lots of fresh parsley. It makes a one-pot meal if you add legumes or nuts, or use it as a side dish for fish or poultry. Quinoa is good in grain-based salads too.

What's the best breakfast cereal?

The one you make yourself. The best way to get a super-nutritious high-fibre breakfast cereal with no added sugar and salt is to create your own. Making your own muesli takes only minutes, unless you prefer your oats toasted. All you do is mix together the following:

- *Traditional rolled oats*. You can also include some rolled barley or rolled rye if you like.
- *Dried fruit* like raisins, sultanas or cranberries, or chopped apricots, dates, figs, peaches or pears.
- *Sunflower seeds and pepitas*.
- *Hazelnut* and/or *ground almond meal*.
- A little powdered *cinnamon* or *nutmeg*.

If you prefer a toasted version, toast the oats, barley and rye by spreading them on an ungreased baking sheet for about 10–15 minutes at 180 degrees Celcius, making sure they don't burn. Cool before mixing with the other ingredients.

This makes a great breakfast at home or to take to work (try soaking it the night before in a little freshly squeezed orange juice).

Taking your pulses

Although we've embraced a few aspects of a healthy Mediterranean diet like good tomatoes, basil and olive oil, we've been slower to latch on to other ingredients like lentils, beans and chickpeas. But, like wholegrains, legumes (or pulses) have serious benefits for women at midlife:

- Because they contain *fibre* as well as other substances called sterols, legumes can reduce blood cholesterol. One US study found that people who ate pulses four or more times a week had a 22 per cent lower risk of coronary heart disease than those who ate them once a week or less.
- Beans, especially black beans and red kidney beans, are a rich source of *antioxidants*, and there's something about soybeans – possibly a plant hormone called genistein – that may explain why countries with a high intake of soy have lower rates of hormone-related cancers like breast and prostate.
- A study coordinated by Monash University in Melbourne following the health of people over 70 in Japan, Sweden, Australia and

Greece for seven years found that those who ate the most legumes were the most likely to live the longest.

* They make it easy to eat more *fibre*. For a healthy gut you need around 30 g of fibre a day, and just one cup of cooked lentils will give you around 15 g.

* They are a slowly digested *carbohydrate* that helps keep blood sugar levels even.

Legumes have fed the world's poor for centuries – and can now help us fend off diseases of affluence. They appear on menus all over the world dressed up in lots of exotic ways; tofu (from soybeans) in Asia; falafel and hummus (from chickpeas) in the Middle East; lentil curries in India; bean and rice dishes in Latin America; and comfort food like minestrone and other bean soups from Italy.

With no tradition of eating pulses, unless you count baked beans, many Australians haven't a clue how to use them. Although dried pulses need cooking and soaking, canned pulses are real convenience food. With a few cans of chickpeas, beans or lentils on hand, you've always got the makings of an easy protein-rich, low fat meal that's low cost too. You can upgrade a bottled pasta sauce with drained, canned lentils and a few vegetables, or add drained chickpeas to sautéed vegetables for a sauce for cous cous, rice, bulgur or quinoa. As for dried red lentils, they're the fast food of the legume world – because they cook in around 15 minutes and don't need soaking, you can turn them into dinner in the time it takes to get a pizza delivered.

If you're after other ways to take your pulses, spread hummus on bread instead of butter or margarine, or give salads more protein and fibre by adding canned, drained pulses.

What about the fart factor?

Wind is less of a problem if you:

* Increase your intake of pulses slowly

- Throw out the soaking water before you cook dried beans
- Include more lentils and chickpeas, as they contain less of the indigestible sugars that can cause wind.

Tips for using pulses.

- While you have to plan ahead to cook with dried beans (i.e. soak them for around 12 hours and then cook them), cooking and freezing a lot at once means they're always there when you need them. It's worth a try – canned pulses are good – but soups, curries and other dishes made by cooking soaked chickpeas and cannelini beans are even better.
- Always drain and rinse canned legumes.
- Most canned legumes are good in salads – even better if you marinate them in dressing for an hour or so before they go in the salad bowl.

Legumes 101

Red lentils Makes great comfort food like dahl, soup or mash.

Green or brown lentils The dried ones need no soaking. Brown lentils are also available canned. Good for soup. Canned lentils add a peppery flavour and texture to salads.

Chickpeas (garbanzos) Available canned or dried. Really versatile – a base for making hummus, to add to curries or use in a vegetarian sauce for cous cous, bulgur or rice.

Cannelini (or great northern beans) Available canned or dried. Good in soups. Marinate with chopped, ripe tomato, olive oil and basil in salads or piled on to toasted bread.

Black beans Available canned or dried. Smaller and sweeter than most legumes, they're a Latin American staple with a smooth velvety texture that makes them good comfort food. A great topping for rice or a filling for burritos if you mix them with sautéed onion, chilli, tomato and sweet corn (canned or fresh) tossed in. Like most legumes, you need to soak them first if you're cooking from scratch, but they're increasingly available canned. Black beans also pack a big nutritional punch – they're as rich in antioxidants as grapes and cranberries.

Red kidney beans Available canned or dried. Add to sauces for rice or pasta or in salads – they go well with chilli and cumin.

The healthy fast food kitchen

Some fine tuning in the kitchen makes it easier to create healthy food fast – especially at dinner.

Essential equipment

You can fill your kitchen with a million gadgets, but unless they're functional – meaning they save time and are easy to clean – they're just more work. The following are good to have:

A SHARP KNIFE

You'll be surprised how much time you save with a sharp stainless steel knife that slices effortlessly through vegetables. To keep it sharp, ask a specialist knife shop or friendly butcher to sharpen it for you. Crushing garlic? Use the flat blade of your kitchen knife to smash each bulb – no fiddly garlic crusher to clean.

SHARP KITCHEN SCISSORS

Faster than a knife for snipping herbs (except basil which is better torn), shallots, trimming the ends of snow peas and beans.

A WOK

Stir-fries with vegetables and a little lean meat, chicken or tofu make short work of midweek dinners.

A STEAMER

Steaming is a fast, no-mess way to cook vegetables that retains more nutrients and flavour. There's no good reason to boil veg – it just wastes nutrients, water, and energy. Compared to steaming, boiling uses more time and fuel. Using a saucepan with a steamer basket, you can have a bowl of lightly cooked vegetables drizzled with vinaigrette, white balsamic vinegar or tamari on the table in minutes. With a two-tier stove-top steamer, you can steam poultry or fish fillets wrapped in foil on the lower tier and add the vegetables to the top tier for the last few minutes of steaming.

MORTAR AND PESTLE
A low-tech way to crush spices together for a curry or to crush nuts to add to a salad dressing or salad.

BLENDER OR FOOD PROCESSOR
To puree vegetables to make healthy soups, dips, sauces and pesto, as well as smoothies.

A RICE COOKER
Non-essential, but it saves time. Rice cookers are easy to clean, turn themselves off when the rice is cooked and keep the rice warm, leaving you free to get on with other things. Also good for cooking rice at weekends to use throughout the week.

LEMON ZESTER
Using grated lemon zest is a quick way to add flavour to salads, desserts, yogurt, fish, dips and muffins.

FOOD CONTAINERS WITH SECURE LIDS
For taking portable breakfasts, lunches and snacks to work.

Food preparation – make it faster

PEEL NOTHING
It's fiddly, and a fast way to lose a lot of nutrients from vegetables and fruit. Many of them are concentrated just under the skin and most fruit and veg have an edible peel.

CHOOSE VEGETABLES THAT NEED MINIMAL, OR ZERO, PREPARATION

Think rocket, baby spinach or salad sprouts. Broccolini, whole baby carrots, button mushrooms, asparagus or bok choy need only washing before tossing into a steamer (yes, you can steam a mushroom). No time to peel and chop an onion? Use kitchen scissors to snip a few shallots. Beans, celery, sugar snap peas or snow peas are other snippable, no-chop vegetables. You can cut them directly into a wok or steamer.

AVOID CLUTTER AND CHAOS

You need a clear working space and to be able to find the tools you need quickly.

WHENEVER YOU MAKE A SOUP OR A CURRY

Try to make enough to freeze some for later.

PUT RECIPES WHERE YOU CAN USE THEM

Instead of clipping a new recipe for a fast, healthy dish and burying it, stick it on the wall above the kitchen bench. If it's instantly visible, you're more likely to shop for the ingredients and try it.

Lighten up – making recipes skinnier and healthier

You don't have to follow recipes to the letter. You can replace carbs with vegetables, use less oil or sugar, replace processed meat with vegetarian alternatives and go easy on the cheese. These adjustments can subtract kilojoules and saturated fat from a dish and pump up its nutrient value.

Fewer carbs – more veg. You can reduce the amount of carbs (like pasta and rice) in dishes by using extra vegetables – you don't lose the comfort factor but you gain more nutrients and fibre by replacing one third or even half of the rice/pasta with vegetables .

* When you're making a risotto or pilaf, reduce the amount of rice and add more chopped vegetables like extra onion, capsicum,

celery, zucchini, mushroom, carrot, pumpkin or add some corn kernels or peas. The same goes for pasta dishes. When you make pasta with pesto, sauté some broccoli and/or cauliflower with shallots, garlic and a little chilli while the pasta cooks. (Or if time's short, just steam the broccoli and cauliflower.) Fold the cooked vegetables in with drained pasta and coat the lot with pesto.

* If you are making pasta or rice salad, use less pasta and rice and more vegetables.
* Only use sheets of lasagne on the top and bottom of a lasagne. If you want you can add a middle layer of eggplant or sliced zucchini.

USING LESS OIL, SUGAR OR SALT

You can often get away with using less oil either for sautéing vegetables for a curry or pasta sauce, for instance, or for baking cakes.

* If a recipe calls for sautéing in ½ cup of oil, I use ¼ or ⅓ of a cup and add more only if I need it.
* Making pesto? Try using less oil than the recipe suggests.
* With cake recipes, I often reduce the amount of fat by substituting half the oil with reduced fat milk or soy milk, and it's usually okay. With desserts and cakes you can often reduce the amount of sugar (especially with US recipes that can be heavy-handed with sugar), i.e. if a recipe calls for two cups of sugar, try using one and a half cups. If it's one cup of sugar, try cutting it to ¾. Adding spices like cinnamon and nutmeg will boost the flavour too.

MAKING LIGHT OF CREAM

* Substitute reduced fat plain yoghurt or buttermilk for sour cream – Vaalia low fat or Attiki reduced fat plain yoghurts are particularly creamy.
* If a recipe includes cream, try reduced fat milk instead.
* For dishes with coconut milk, substitute light coconut milk (less

saturated fat and kilojoules). But the amount of saturated fat can vary between brands – compare labels to find the lightest.

WHAT TO USE INSTEAD OF BACON

❋ Bacon and ham often turn up in recipes as a flavour booster. But they're hardly a health food, so use mushrooms instead – they have a meaty texture and strong flavour that works. Better still, they're useful for weight control – a study from Johns Hopkins Bloomberg School of Public Health found that using mushrooms instead of meat can actually boost a meal's filling power – and reduce a meal's kilojoule content at the same time.

GO EASY ON THE CHEESE

❋ Cheese tastes wonderful and has the added benefit of being rich in calcium – but it's also rich in saturated fat and high in kilojoules. A smarter way to eat it is to use strong flavoured cheeses (like fetta, parmesan, romano or goat's cheese) as flavour enhancers in dishes rather than as a major ingredient. Try a little crumbled reduced fat fetta or a few small pieces of goat's cheese added to a salad; a little Parmesan added to risotto or pesto; reduced fat fetta added to bean dishes. The amount of saturated fat in different brands of fetta cheese can vary quite a lot, so compare the label to find the lightest.

Eat out – eat fit

You can choose your friends, but you can't always choose where they want to eat! It was a Friday night and we were asked to join friends at an Italian place where we'd never eaten before – and which clearly knew nothing of the Mediterranean Diet. There was grilled fish but it was served with chips. There was bruschetta, but so sodden with olive oil you could have picked it up and wrung it out. Apart from that it was hard to find anything that wasn't crumbed, deep fried or finished with cream.

If you have a choice, it makes sense to eat in a restaurant where there's lean food on the menu. If in doubt, ask to see a menu or ring up before you go.

* *Don't be scared to ask if the chef can lighten a dish up a bit.* Ask for fish that's grilled instead of fried, vegetables or a salad instead of chips, or less cheese and more vegetables on a pizza.

* *Be aware that eating out with other people tends to make you eat more.* The more people sitting around a table, the more you're likely to eat. Be conscious of the crowd effect, and don't cave in to pressure to eat or drink more. Sharing dishes can be another problem with group eating – if you're the only one who's chosen something healthy, you can end up with only a fraction of your dish and having to fill up on high fat foods you're trying to avoid. Remember, it's okay to opt not to share if you're eating in a group.

* *Find out more about what you're ordering.* Is the fish grilled, fried or baked? What's in the pasta sauce? (Tomato-based sauces are generally lower in kilojoules and saturated fat.) Is there coconut milk in the curry? (Coconut milk is high in saturated fat.)

* *Be guided by your appetite.* Don't feel that because you're eating out, you should eat three courses. If main courses are large, you may need nothing else besides a side salad. Or two entrees may be enough. Pasta dishes and risottos can be really generous – you may be better off with an entree size and a mixed salad as your main course.

* *Order plain bread* rather than garlic or herb bread.

* *Order water* and you'll drink less alcohol.

* *Choose a skinnier cuisine.* Japanese, Thai and Vietnamese usually have good options, but if you're unsure how something's cooked, ask. Dishes that can be high in saturated fat include tempura (deep-fried in batter) and anything cooked in coconut milk.

❋ *Never assume 'vegetarian' on the menu translates as 'less saturated fat' or low in kilojoules.* Some healthy sounding vegetarian dishes can be deep-fried or made with pastry, or both. Find out what you're ordering first.

Eat healthier at work too

If you work in a city, chances are you're surrounded by a plethora of lunch options. Avoid temptation and a depleted bank account by:

MAKING A HABIT OF BRINGING LUNCH

Pack lunch the night before and include some protein – fish, tofu, nuts, legumes, egg, low fat yoghurt or low fat cheese or lean meat, with vegetables and some healthy carbs to help you last the distance.

KEEPING A STASH OF HEALTHY SNACKS

A supply of fruit, nuts, dried fruit, trail mix or low fat yoghurt at work means you've always got healthy food when you need it. If there's a freezer, you can keep some good wholegrain rolls or fruit bread too.

CHALLENGING THE CAKE CULTURE

There's nothing wrong with sharing a birthday cake, but it's hard to stick to a healthy eating plan if cake, biscuits and fundraiser chocolate are always on offer at work. The obvious strategy is to just say no, but you could lead by example and do something different for your own birthday, like bring in a plate of exotic fruit to share instead of cake, or bake a healthier cake yourself.

DRINKING WATER THROUGHOUT THE DAY

Keep a bottle on your desk; often the urge to eat something is a signal to drink water.

Action list

- Set aside time for some product research in the supermarket – compare labels and figure out which foods are the healthiest buy. This helps you make informed choices faster on your regular shopping trips.

- Clean out the cupboard and fridge and make room for healthier foods.

- Not used to cooking with legumes? Find a curry recipe using lentils or canned chickpeas and try it out.

- Add some vegetables to the weekend big breakfast.

Chapter 7

The shape stealers

For many women, the mid-40s onwards coincides with job success – you might have reached a point in your career where you earn more and have a lifestyle that includes more eating out, more glasses of wine – and more kilojoules. If this also coincides with a busy job that makes it hard to be physically active, you've got a recipe for weight gain.

There's no shortage of ways to camouflage a ballooning mid-section – just ask Trinny and Susannah. You could take refuge in a suit or a long jacket, concealing the sides of your body. A long enough jacket means no one can see that your waist no longer goes in at the sides. There are loose shirts, caftans and all that contoured underwear in the lingerie department that lift and flatten the drooping, pouchy bits. But in the end when you peel off your clothes your potbelly is still where you left it.

Not that this is all about vanity – if you're scanning clothes racks for tops to camouflage an expanding mid-section, remember that wardrobe problems aren't the worst thing about packing on weight round your waist. As mentioned earlier, it's not great for your long-term health either. A couple of extra kilos are no drama, but if you're creeping towards a waist measurement of 80 cm or more, you're also heading towards an increased risk of problems like heart disease, diabetes, breast and bowel cancer and gall stones.

That's why it's good to think of menopause as a kind of wake up call – a message from your body that there are changes afoot and it's time to take more care of yourself.

Why alcohol goes to your waistline as well as your head

If alcohol were as chewy as apples, it'd be hard to drink as much as we do. But the stuff slips down and if you're sharing a bottle of wine with dinner, then by the time the bill arrives you've added around 1200 kilojoules – the equivalent of a serve of French fries or a Snickers Bar on top of dinner. This is no big deal if it's happening once or twice a week, but if you're regularly averaging two drinks or more each night, the kilojoules add up – especially if you're drinking spirits and adding sugary soft drinks as mixers.

But aside from its kilojoule content, the other pitfall with alcohol is that too much skews your judgement – any resolve to eat the entree size pasta dish instead of the main, or skip the profiteroles for dessert, can melt away after one Merlot too many.

There's nothing wrong with drinking in moderation – two standard drinks or less daily keeps you within the low risk level of drinking for women. But if you're drinking more, there are good reasons to ease up now, and avoiding hot flushes is one of them – alcohol is a common trigger.

Along with the kilojoule load, another effect of overdoing alcohol regularly is that it can sap your energy levels, something you may not recognise until you've experienced a few alcohol free days and realised how much sparkier you feel after an alcohol free night. And the more energy you have, the more you'll feel like fitting a walk into your day.

If you feel tired after a long day at work, don't count on a glass of wine to give you a lift. Blood sugar drops between 4 pm and 6 pm and having a drink to perk you up, as some women do, can actually slow you down. Given that alcohol can have a sedative effect, you're better off with fruit juice.

Do you often drink after work when you get home?

There's nothing wrong with this unless you have too many refills. But it's also good to find other ways to unwind after work. That way, your brain doesn't learn to associate relaxing (or coping with stress) with pouring a drink. Try to change the ritual – go for a walk or sit down with a different kind of drink.

Do you always drink when you go out?

Try not drinking at all sometimes. You might be surprised to find how much you can enjoy yourself without it – and again it helps break that mental connection that links going out to having to drink. If that's too hard, decide how many drinks you'll have and stick to it. Avoid shouts – it's easier to control your alcohol intake when you're drinking at your own pace, not someone else's, and alternate alcoholic drinks with water.

When less is more

Drinking less helps keep your tolerance down. It helps you enjoy the effects of alcohol with fewer drinks and fewer kilojoules. Increasing the number of drinks over time gradually increases your tolerance of alcohol so you need more and more to have an effect.

'I'm drinking less but still enjoying it – it only takes one drink for me to feel an effect whereas it used take four,' says 50-year-old Jo, a Sydney caterer whose habit of drinking four or more vodkas each night began in her 20s. Since finishing the Australian Centre for Addiction Research's Controlled Drinking Program, she's cut down to two glasses of wine five nights a week.

'But if I slip up and drink three glasses instead, I have nothing the following day,' she adds. 'I used to have a drink as soon as I got home from work. Now I don't pour a drink until I've done everything.'

Do other people pressure you to drink?

I have a theory about this and it also applies to people who pressure you to eat more than you want: it helps them feel better about their own habits.

Stick to your guns and remember that how much you drink is your choice, not someone else's. One of the benefits of getting older is that it gets so much easier to stand your ground and not be swayed by what

'I realised that drinking had just become a habit – I'd have a glass of wine while I was cooking dinner and then more wine when I was eating, then I'd sit down with my partner to watch TV and we'd have a couple more drinks,' says 48-year-old Sarah. 'But I realised it was just something we did while we watched TV and I needed to find something else to do. Now I cut up some fresh fruit and nibble on that instead.'

'I'd open a bottle of wine when I got home from work and keep drinking – I think it was partly because my husband does shift work and I'm alone in the evenings. But it was getting harder to recover in the mornings, and I also knew I had to lose weight – a bottle of wine was a lot of calories I didn't need,' says Sandra, a 50-year-old financial adviser. 'Now I don't drink at all – and feel much better in the mornings. I use the evenings to go for a walk or go to the gym.'

'What's been interesting since I stopped drinking is that when I'm out with other people I get the sense that some people are actually envious that I don't need to drink,' Sandra says.

Women like Sarah and Sandra aren't unusual, says Professor Sitharthan Thiagarajan of the Australian Centre for Addiction Research in Sydney, which runs a free program available by correspondence or online that helps people learn to drink less and drink more slowly.

'They finish work, come home, open a bottle and start drinking. If they're drinking from a cask, which isn't transparent like a bottle, it's much harder to keep track of how many drinks they're having, and often they drink too fast,' he says. 'They're not necessarily dependent on alcohol, they just need help to control how much they drink.'

other people think. But if you find it difficult, use other strategies like saying you can't drink because you're taking antibiotics, or you can fill your glass with something that looks like alcohol, like cranberry juice – but you shouldn't *have* to justify not drinking.

How much can you really drink?
Alcohol and the gender gap

It's Saturday night and a woman and her partner are each sipping a glass of wine while they order dinner in a restaurant. Both are drinking the same amount of alcohol, but the odds are that by the time the entree appears and each glass is empty, her blood alcohol concentration will be higher than his.

If there's one area where there's no gender equality, it's alcohol. A woman's body has less water and more fat than a man's. As a result, any alcohol she drinks is less diluted. Size matters too. Women tend to be smaller and alcohol is more concentrated in a smaller body mass.

Compared to men, women also tend to have less of an enzyme (alcohol dehydrogenase, or ADH) that breaks down alcohol. This means more alcohol enters their blood stream, and may contribute to a higher risk of liver and brain damage. Drinking more than two standard drinks daily, and in particular frequently drinking four standard drinks a day or more, will increase this risk.

Developing alcohol problems appears to be telescoped for women. Compared to men, they can become more intoxicated and develop more serious problems earlier in their drinking careers.

Why not shop around for lower alcohol wine?

We're used to checking food labels, why not wine as well? Although many Australian wines, especially red, contain 14–15 per cent alcohol, others are only 10 or 11 per cent or, in some cases, lower still. Some are naturally lower in alcohol than others. Hunter Valley semillons are one example, with alcohol contents often as low as 10 or 11 per cent. Generally, the cooler the temperature of the wine-growing area, the lower the alcohol content. Riesling from Tasmania, Sauvignon Blanc from the Adelaide Hills and Pinot Noir from Gippsland and the

What's a standard drink?

Checking the label on the bottle, can or cask tells you how many standard drinks it contains, e.g. a bottle of spirits contains 22 standard drinks and a bottle of wine around 7.5 (though it depends on the alcohol content of the wine – a bottle of wine with a lower alcohol content will contain more standard drinks than one with a higher alcohol content). The number of standard drinks in pre-mixed drinks can vary. Make sure you read the label.

Wine A standard drink is smaller than you think – just 100 ml. But some wine glasses are so large, it's not hard to pour a drink that's actually 200 ml. An average serve poured in a bar is around 150 ml – one and a half standard drinks.

Spirits A 30 ml nip or a shot of spirits is one standard drink – a single cocktail can be a few standard drinks in one hit, depending on how many nips are used.

Beer A 375 ml can or bottle of full strength beer contains 1.5 standard drinks; a 375 ml can or bottle of light beer is just 0.8 of a standard drink.

Mornington Peninsula also tend to be lighter – just check the label to read the percentage of alcohol. If you like something sweeter, there's moscato, the light, fruity Italian style white that can be as low as 5.5 per cent alcohol.

Alcohol and women's health – some good news and some bad.

Alcohol and bones. Too many glasses can promote thinning bones. The problem seems to be that alcohol inhibits the normal formation of new bones.

Alcohol and mood. Despite its party drug reputation, too much alcohol may give you the blues. If that conjures up images of people drowning their sorrows or using alcohol to lift a blue mood, that's not always the case. For some people, alcohol comes first and depression comes later. No one really knows why – the guess is that alcohol may affect the part of the brain that controls mood – but research by the Australian Centre for Addiction Research suggests that when people learn to control their alcohol consumption and drink less, their mood improves.

Alcohol and cancer. We've all heard that alcohol, in small amounts, can be heart-healthy, but the message that alcohol is also linked to an increased risk of cancer has been slower to trickle through. According to the World Cancer Research Fund, there's convincing evidence that alcohol contributes to breast cancer – recent US research has found that drinking between one and two alcoholic drinks daily can increase the risk of breast cancer by 10 per cent, compared with women who average less than one drink daily – but the risk jumps to 30 per cent for women drinking more than three drinks a day. If you do drink, it's all the more reason to load up on wholegrains, leafy green vegetables and oranges. Foods rich in the B vitamin folate may help counteract the harmful effects of alcohol on the breasts. More than two drinks a day may also slightly raise the risk of endometrial cancer. The reason for the link with both breast and endometrial cancer may be that alcohol raises oestrogen levels. Alcohol probably contributes to bowel cancer in women too, suggests the World Cancer Research Fund.

Alcohol and the heart. A little alcohol of any kind can be good for the arteries, as it relaxes the artery walls. Wine also contains heart-healthy antioxidants. But the key here is moderation. Too many drinks contribute to high blood pressure that in turn increases heart disease risk.

Alcohol and skin. Thanks to less active oil glands, skin has a habit of drying out as you get older. Given that alcohol can have a dehydrating effect on skin, that's another reason to go easy.

Alcohol and the female brain. It's nice to know that research from the US Nurses' Health Study shows that older women who average one drink per day have a 20 per cent lower risk of impaired thinking, compared to non-drinkers. This may be for the same reason that a little alcohol is good for the heart too – it helps arteries stay healthy, improving blood flow to the brain. The flipside of this is that women's brains are more vulnerable than men's to too much alcohol. Alcohol abuse can shrink the part of the brain that's linked to learning and memory, and some research suggests women are more susceptible to this than men.

The new weight loss enhancer – more sleep

Just imagine walking into your local health food store and buying a pill that not only improved performance but kept your immune system healthy and helped prevent weight gain too – we'd buy bottles of the stuff! But we all have free access to something that has the same effect, if you can get it: eight hours sleep a night.

You'd think that spending less time asleep and more time awake would be a recipe for burning up more kilojoules and losing weight, but that's not how it works. Too little sleep seems to go hand in hand with too many kilos. A decade or so ago, when researchers started noticing a link between night shift workers and weight gain, the cause was thought to be that people ate more to try to stay awake. But there's more to it than that. Supposedly, the chronic lack of sleep can disrupt the hormones that regulate hunger, explains Dr Naomi Rogers, a researcher with the Woolcock Institute of Medical Research in Sydney. If you're regularly short-changed on sleep, up go levels of a hormone called grehlin that stimulates your appetite, and down go levels of leptin, another hormone that tells your body when you've stored enough fat and don't need more to eat. This wouldn't be so bad if these surges of 'hungry' hormone made you crave a nice bowl of steamed vegetables or a crisp apple, but as most of us know – and some research bears this out – fatigue is more likely to make you want muffins or more of the leftover birthday cake in the office. When we're tired we tend to eat more (and more of the wrong stuff) to try to stay alert, and we have less energy to exercise. Lack of sleep can also make you feel stressed – and stress can make us eat more too.

Given that people now sleep on average an hour less at night than they did 50 years ago and have also gained more weight at the same time has led some researchers to suspect the two trends may be connected. Too little sleep may be one of the factors that conspire to make us fatter. The US Nurses' Heath Study, which has followed the health of thousands of women over decades, has found that those who sleep the least gain the most weight.

But when it comes to getting the right amount of sleep, being female is a disadvantage all by itself. For reasons that experts can't fully explain, women tend to have more insomnia than men – one theory is that we're programmed for lighter sleep so we're more alert to sounds of crying babies and children. This would be okay if nature gave us a break from this once we've kissed our reproductive years goodbye, but the problem has a habit of getting worse at midlife – sleep disruption is one of the most common problems reported by women moving into menopause.

Shifting hormones in the run-up to menopause and after can make it harder to get to sleep and make women more susceptible to disturbed sleep, according to the National Sleep Foundation in the US. Hot flushes or night sweats, side effects of hormonal changes, are common culprits.

To find out if changing hormone levels around menopause could affect women's sleep quality, researchers asked 630 women aged 43 to 53 to keep a sleep diary over the course of a single menstrual cycle. They found that, compared to women who were still pre-menopausal, women who already had early signs of menopause were more likely to have disturbed sleep.

STRESS

Worrying about work and/or family matters can have you lying awake at night, your mind churning with thoughts about money, relationships, troubled kids and looming deadlines. Too little time and too much to do often mean there's not enough down-time before you go to bed, making it hard to unwind and fall asleep.

PARENTHOOD

Kids who've turned into teenagers can be powerful sleep disrupters – either because it's past 1 am and they're still not home, or because you have to pick them up from somewhere at midnight.

ALCOHOL

While alcohol does a great job of helping you doze off quickly, drinking too much too close to bedtime can sometimes backfire. One drink might be okay, but too much can fragment your sleep because of falling blood alcohol levels that can wake you up later in the night.

NICOTINE

There are a zillion reasons to avoid nicotine – keeping you awake is one of them.

While the odd sleepless night is no big deal, chronic sleep deprivation can interfere with the way your body regulates blood sugar, increasing the risk of developing diabetes. It can even make you more susceptible to infection. When researchers from the University of Chicago gave the flu vaccine to sleep-deprived students, their immune systems produced only half the normal number of antibodies to the vaccine.

There are links between lack of sleep and heart disease too – one of them is that lack of sleep can increase the risk of high blood pressure.

In 2003, a US study of 71,000 women – again, part of Harvard University's Nurses Health Study – reported that both too little sleep (seven hours or less), and too much (more than eight hours) appeared to raise the risk of heart disease.

A good night's sleep is no luxury. It's what your body needs to repair its tissues and replenish the hormones that make it work. Yet sleep deprivation often goes unrecognised because people don't make the connection between feeling lethargic and irritable during the day and lack of sleep.

People can get used to sleep deprivation and it's often not until they experience how great they feel having slept well that they realise the effect lack of sleep has. They also feel more like doing exercise when they get enough sleep, and when you exercise you sleep better.

But along with demands on our time, another enemy of sleep is the idea that functioning on a few hours sleep is a sign of I-can-do-anything heroism, while needing eight hours means you're a feeble wimp. As our lives have sped up and become fuller, cutting down on sleep time has been seen as a way to do more and improve performance. The reality is that it can make you less effective – not to mention add a couple of years to your face.

Allow yourself at least an hour to relax before bedtime

If you can't get to sleep when your head hits the pillow, perhaps you haven't allowed yourself enough time to unwind before bedtime. If you're on the go all day, the moment you climb into bed could be the first quiet time you've had, and your mind can buzz with things to do and remember.

'Until I got into my mid-40s, I was the kind of person who went to bed, put her head on the pillow and slept through until morning. But I honestly think my problem with sleep was more my family than my hormones,' says 51-year-old Natalie. 'I'd wake up in the night and find it hard to get back to sleep again either because the kids were staying up late studying and I'd hear them moving around downstairs, or I'd hear them coming home late from a party. Maybe I'd just become a lighter sleeper but, whatever the reason, if something woke me up I'd find it hard to get back to sleep again. The worse thing was that a bad night's sleep would make me feel anxious about getting enough sleep the next night. If I woke up in the middle of the night, the anxiety of feeling I might not get enough sleep would keep me awake.'

Eventually Natalie worked out a few strategies that, most of the time, improved her sleep. 'Switching on the ceiling fan really worked – the noise of the fan blotted out any other sound so I was less likely to wake up. I also read up on relaxation techniques and tried some of them out when I couldn't get back to sleep. The one that works best for me is one of the simplest. You make your left shoulder go heavy and limp and say to yourself "my left shoulder is heavy". Then you do the same thing on your right side. You just keep repeating "my left side is heavy, my right side is heavy" until you fall asleep. Most of the time it works for me – I think it's because focusing on repeating the words stops my mind racing.'

Why can't I sleep?

A couple of sleepless nights can also cause sleep anxiety – meaning you can't sleep for worrying that you'll have another sleepless night. If you're not asleep after 20 minutes, the advice is to get up and go to another room for a while and then try again. This advice applies any time you can't sleep: getting out of bed is important, because if you stay there, you're inadvertently training yourself to stay awake in bed. Lying there worrying can also increase your levels of stress hormones, making it even harder to get to sleep.

How about pills to help you sleep?

ON PRESCRIPTION

Prescription drugs like benzodiazepines have their place for the occasional sleepless night, to help you cope with jet lag or for short-term help with grief. But taking them continuously for more than two weeks can make you develop a tolerance to them. This can mean the pills don't work as well and it may become even harder to get to sleep – a condition called rebound insomnia.

OVER THE COUNTER

Valerian is a common ingredient in herbal sleep remedies, but studies of its effectiveness are mixed. Some research suggests that 400–900 mg at bedtime improves sleep quality and reduces the time it takes to fall asleep, but a study from the University of California found it was no better than a placebo. An Ayurvedic herb called *withania somnifera* (also known as winter cherry or Indian ginseng) is also used as a sleep inducer but you should get a therapeutic dose prescribed by a good herbalist rather than self-prescribing (contact The National Herbalists' Association of Australia on (02) 8765 0071, or the Australian National Therapists' Association on 1800 817 577). Melatonin supplements may help you get over jet lag, but may not work for insomnia. Other over-the-counter remedies are based on sedating anti-histamines but, again, prolonged use isn't recommended as they can make you drowsy during the day.

I've tried everything and I still can't sleep

If you've exhausted all possibilities, your GP can refer you to a hospital sleep clinic. If the suspect is obstructive sleep apnoea, a problem affecting breathing during sleep that causes daytime fatigue and sleepines, you need a sleepover in a sleep laboratory They will monitor your brain-waves, breathing, heart rate and oxygen levels. If you have insomnia, you don't usually need a sleep study, but could be referred to an insomnia clinic for help with strategies to help you get a good night's sleep.

How to get a better night's sleep.

Reset your brain clock. Your brain clock is a cluster of brain cells in the hypothalamus that determines your sleep/wake time and is regulated by light and darkness, explains Delwyn Bartlett, a sleep psychologist with the Woolcock Institute of Medical Research in Sydney. Here's how to keep it on track:

Wake up at the same time every morning, even on weekends. This is more important than going to bed at the same time every night.

'Going to bed doesn't guarantee sleep if you're anxious or stressed and paying too much attention to your sleep,' Delwyn says. 'Sleep needs to be something you do without thinking about it. Waking up at the same time cues your brain to release sleep/wake hormones at the right time.'

Get the light right. Melatonin, the sleep hormone that gets your brain ready for sleep, needs diminishing levels of light to help it kick in. Sitting under bright light or staring at your laptop can delay its effects. Keep lights in the bedroom low before you go to sleep. Once you turn out the light, make sure there's no other light source in the room. Even small 'on' lights from computers or televisions can be disturbing for some people. If the alarm clock has a light, turn it away from you. Have curtains that let you wake up to morning light (unless you're working shifts).

Keep the bedroom serene. A calm, uncluttered bedroom can go a long way to making you feel more relaxed when you finally climb into bed. Banish anything related to work from your bedroom, and try to keep it tidy – having stuff strewn everywhere is just another reminder of the things you have to do.

Check your blankets. To feel sleepy, your body temperature needs to fall. An overheated bedroom or an electric blanket turned up too high can make it hard to sleep. But a warm bath an hour before bed can help your temperature fall. The warm water artificially raises your temperature that then has to come down once you're out of the bath.

Think about what you drink and eat before bedtime. Drinks containing caffeine – coffee, tea, cocoa, green tea and cola – can keep you awake. Although caffeine's stimulant effect is strongest in the first hour or so after taking it, it can still be in your system eight hours later. Eat earlier rather than later. If you have dinner at 9 pm, your body will still be trying to digest it when you're in bed, and will be keeping you awake. It's better to have dinner earlier and eat something light before bed if you're hungry. A late dinner also means you're less likely to feel like food the next morning – but skip breakfast and you're more likely to raid the office cookie jar later in the morning. If you're wanting a good bedtime snack, aim for something light and easy to digest that includes carbohydrates – low fat warm milk or some soy milk, a piece of wholegrain toast, a banana or a fruit smoothie.

Create a sound barrier. Noise can interrupt your sleep even though you don't remember it the next morning. Ear plugs can help, as can 'white noise', which means using some sounds (a fan for example) to mask other, more disturbing noises – the fan can also help cool you down if you overheat.

Have a snore refuge. I'd never suggest couples sleep in separate rooms BUT having a spare room to retreat to occasionally when your sleep is broken because he's snoring or you're overheating – or both – can really help.

Get regular exercise. Being physically active can help you get a better night's sleep. Just don't do it too close to bedtime. Exercise is an energiser and it can perk you up and make it hard to nod off. On the other hand, some experts suggest that the dip in temperature that comes five hours or so after a late afternoon workout can help you sleep.

Action list

- Count how many drinks you have each day – remember to count standard drinks, not just the number of glasses. If it's often more than two, think about how you can cut down.

- Try a lower alcohol wine.

- Banish anything related to work from your bedroom.

- Try to allow at least one hour's 'down' time before you go to bed.

Conclusion

Making it happen

long with eating and exercise, there's a third element to
keeping your body fit and firm – your attitude. 'Both men
and women take on weight loss as a war, but with men it's
Desert Storm, an all out, take-no-prisoners war, and with women it can
be the Hundred Years' War – a long protracted battle that alternates attack with retreat and negotiations.'

I wish I could take the credit for this great quote, but it was a
memorable comment from nutritionist Karen Miller-Kovach, the
scientific adviser to Weight Watchers in the US, making the point that
while men tend to tackle weight loss in a direct, no-nonsense way, for
many women it can be a more complex, tortured process. For one thing,
women's relationship with food can be more emotional, especially if
they use food to cope with stress or feelings. Some women find it very
difficult to resist certain foods – then when they succumb, they feel
guilty, and this encourages them to eat more.

For this and other reasons, the road to getting fitter and firmer isn't
always smooth. You can get stalled on exercise plateaus on the way. There
will be moments when life, work or family – or all three – make it
difficult to stick to a fitness routine. But Australian research from the
Queensland Institute of Technology suggests that self-efficacy – the
belief that you can get the result you want – is a strong factor in helping
women lose weight at midlife.

'Exercise and eating healthier are the two "legs" that help you lose
weight, but a woman's mental attitude is like a third leg, and I think it's

this third leg that dictates how well the other two legs go,' says researcher Rhonda Anderson, whose study of middle-aged women and weight loss found that self-efficacy emerged as a strong influence on a woman's decision to do more exercise or eat healthier food.

'A person with high dietary self-efficacy believes they can eat healthily no matter what – even when bored, upset, tired, on holiday or at a party," says Rhonda. People with high self-efficacy are motivated and optimistic. When the going gets tough, they keep going, she says. On the other hand, people with low self-efficacy are more likely to give up when things get tough.

The good news, she says, is that we can improve our self-efficacy by developing skills, having role models and getting encouragement from others.

Motivation

I've been running for three or four mornings a week for the last 20-odd years, and guess what? On a grey, chilly morning with wind gusts bending the branches of the trees outside, the last thing I want to do is open the door and run into the cold. Even after all these years, a little voice pipes up with a few reasons not to put on my running shoes. 'It's too cold; I'll do it later, I don't have time; the kitchen's a mess – I should clean it; I've got a deadline'. But, mostly, I manage to talk over the little voice and get out there and run.

Once you begin to see and feel the results of regular exercise – a better shape and more energy – you'll grow an inner drive that keeps you motivated. By then you'll be reaping so many benefits that you'll want to keep moving. But during the early weeks while you're still establishing an exercise habit, motivation can be hard. Sometimes you have to grit your teeth and, as the ad says, just do it.

Even if you're committed, there may still be times when, like me, you have to push yourself out of the door, and these are the tactics that can work when you bump into barriers like miserable weather and tight schedules.

- *Decide the greatest benefits you get from working out.* Make a mental list of them (or, better still, write them down and stick them somewhere where you'll see them). Use them to remind yourself when your resolve falters. Keep at it, and it won't be long before these positive thoughts kick in automatically every time you try to talk yourself out of exercising.
- *Schedule exercise* in your diary as you would any other important activity.
- *Connect the benefits of working out* to something that's really meaningful to you rather than something vague like 'it's good for me' or 'I know I should'. For instance, I have this favourite pencil skirt and the reason it looks good is because I keep in shape. When I start thinking of reasons to skip my morning run or walk, I picture myself slipping into the skirt, zipping it up and seeing how good it looks with a flat belly and a firm bum. This works for me. But it's different for everyone. Perhaps it could be something connected to your health. If your blood pressure or cholesterol levels are on the high side, remind yourself that each session of exercise will work towards lowering it.
- *Find a friend.* Research shows that exercising with someone else helps you stay motivated and helps to make sure you turn up for a walk, run or fitball class. It works in two ways – if you've made an arrangement with someone you're more committed, and it's also fun working out when you're catching up with someone.
- Just as you can learn how to talk yourself out of something, you can also learn how to talk yourself *into* it. *Remind yourself that you'll feel energised* after a workout – even on days when you feel tired; that exercise will lift your mood; how good it is to know that your exercise is done for the day.
- *Take practical steps to make it easy.* If a run or a walk is

scheduled for the next morning, have the right clothes and shoes all ready to go the night before. If you go to the gym, keep a gym bag ready to go with clothes, shoes, towel and water bottle so it's always ready to take to work or put in the car.

* *Buy new workout clothes.* A new top won't make you fitter, but having something you feel good in can be an extra incentive to put it on and workout.

* *Reward yourself* with something when you've met your goal – though you may find that the way you feel is reward enough.

* *Don't beat yourself up if you miss a session.* Some people have an all or nothing approach to exercise and eating – they feel if they're not doing everything perfectly, they've blown it. This gets you nowhere. Missing a regular walk or skipping a session at the gym is a hiccup, not a disaster. Put it behind you and pick up again the next day.

Goal setting

Imagining yourself looking slim and well at some future event – say, wearing a pretty dress on Christmas Day with the family – is a great self-efficacy booster. These sorts of pleasant daydreams are not a waste of time; on the contrary, they help you to feel optimistic and purposeful. However, you're more likely to arrive in that happy place if you actually set yourself goals and monitor your progress towards achieving them.

The first thing to do is to write down what it is you want to do. Don't be afraid to admit what it is; go on, be brave! But make sure also that your goals are both specific and realistic. 'I'm going to exercise more' is too vague, and 'I want to start running six kilometres four times a week' is unrealistic. Goals that are more specific and realistic could be: At the end of 10 weeks I want to be able to jog for 20 minutes without stopping;

In three months' time I will be exercising for six hours a week; At the end of the month I'll be walking for 30 minutes a day.

Make it easier for yourself by committing to something like a community walk or running event to take part in, like the Can Too women did. Or you could book a walking/trekking holiday for which you have to get fit.

Make a plan to meet these goals

Create a plan made up of smaller goals to help you reach the big goal and accommodate your increasing fitness.

For instance, to reach the 'In three months' time I will be exercising for six hours a week' goal, have smaller goals, like:

◉ *In one month's time* I'll be exercising for 2 ½ hours a week.
◉ *In two months' time* I'll be exercising for 4 hours a week.
◉ *In three months' time* I'll be exercising 6 hours a week.

Meeting smaller goals along the way gives you a sense of accomplishment that helps you keep going. What this does is establish a positive cycle when you feel satisfaction at meeting a goal, which improves your sense of self-efficacy, which gives you more confidence to set another goal … and on it goes. If your confidence starts to flag, it might help to also write down the skills and strengths you already possess that will get you to where you want to be. Remind yourself of other times when your persistence and patience finally brought rewards and how you have successfully managed lots of other challenging situations in your life. We are more likely to achieve our goals if we also believe in our ability to succeed.

Overcoming exercise blocks

It's boring Try a different kind of exercise – if you're bored on the treadmill, try a boxing class; Exercise with a friend; Change your walking/running route; Listen to music on your iPod or the radio while you run/walk.

I'm tired/I don't feel like it Remind yourself how much better you'll feel when you've finished – and what a sense of accomplishment you'll have.

It's too cold Add some layers that you can peel off as you warm up. Remind yourself how warm you'll feel later. In winter, it's a good idea to sleep in yoga pants and singlet – doing so makes it easier to just grab a jacket and shoes and head out the door.

It's too dark Choose a well lit area to run/walk, stay off the road and wear light-coloured clothing.

I don't have time Think about this for a minute. Ask yourself – do I really not have time or am I just using this as an excuse? If you really, really don't have time, make it a quickie. If you only have 20 minutes, or even ten minutes to workout instead of 30 minutes or an hour, use this time to do something – some brisk hill walking; some strength-training at home; jog for ten minutes and walk for ten; find some stairs and run up and down them a few times and skip for a few minutes. Or do a mini-workout using your own body weight – some lunges or walking lunges, some push-ups, triceps dips and crunches.

I'm bad at sport Me too. But guess what? You can be really bad at sport, but still put one foot in front of another and keep going. Or pick up a weight and keep lifting it.

I'll feel stupid Possibly. But you'll get over it (you're a grown-up, remember). And the chances are that no one is watching you anyway.

'There's always time to exercise,' says Sydney psychologist Susan Nicholson, who averages an hour's swimming, walking or cycling and the occasional run most days of the week. 'People say to me "how do you do it?" but there's always some wasted time that you can use. I think people often think they should stay back for an hour at work, but I think that if they went out and got moving instead they'd be more effective at work. You just have to make it a priority.'

At 50, Susan has just taken up surfing, which she's added to her summer routine of a couple of six-kilometre ocean swims each week and six five-kilometre walks. In winter it's cycling – two 40-kilometre rides each week and four eight-kilometre walks. 'I hate the gym because I don't like being indoors. For me it's about being in a natural outdoor environment. It helps me wind down. I work with a lot of people so I like to have some time alone, away from any mental stuff. She's also practising what she preaches: When she worked as a clinical psychologist, she'd prescribe exercise, preferably in a natural setting, for clients with depression, and found that it got results. Now she consults to companies, teaching senior executives to manage stress.

'I recommend exercise and I notice that with people who don't take it up, their mental performance is less sharp than those who do. The people who exercise also say that not only does it help them manage stress better, they find they have more time because they're more effective.'

When weight loss grinds to a halt

You swapped chips for steamed veggies, joined the gym and the kilos began dropping off – or at least they did to begin with. Then, suddenly, the weight loss honeymoon was over and, despite the better diet and increased activity, the numbers on the scales have stayed the same.

It's known as the weight loss plateau and it's really common – and it can be so disheartening it sends some people back to the couch, convinced that more exercise and a better diet don't work. But it's not all bad news. For one thing, it's normal. Weight loss doesn't always happen in a linear fashion. Some months you might lose one kilo, while in others you might lose three. There are also ways to coax your body into losing more weight. One way is to add strength-training to your fitness routine if you haven't already, or to change the kind of exercise you do – if you're walking, try jogging instead or a cardio class at the gym.

But a really important thing to remember is that even when weight loss has stalled, you're still ahead because you've lost weight, not gained it, and the chances are your health is better for it. For instance, if someone with risk factors for heart disease, diabetes or insulin resistance becomes more active, studies show that their health improves, even if their weight doesn't change.

Changing how you eat can also help reprogram your body into losing weight again. You could try eating more frequently. Try having five smaller meals rather than three large meals through the day. Or you could try increasing the amount of protein you eat and reducing the carbs for a couple of weeks (but aim for healthy wholegrain carbs).

How about eating more? The woman with some of the best credentials for advising on eating and weight loss is Australian scientist Dr Amanda Sainsbury-Salis, an expert in obesity research, who really knows what it's like to struggle with weight – she's now 28 kilos lighter than when she first began using her training as a scientist to solve her own weight problems. Eating too little, she explains, can backfire, causing changes in brain chemistry that make it harder to shed weight.

Research by Sainsbury-Salis, who is now a senior research fellow at the Garvan Institute of Medical Research in Sydney, found that restricting kilojoules could activate brain chemicals that caused metabolism to slow down. If restricting food made metabolism slower, she wondered, could eating more food rev it up again?

Researching the scientific literature, Amanda found studies that suggested the answer was yes. She tested the theory on herself the next time she found herself stuck on a weight loss plateau. But instead of persevering with low kilojoule food, she responded to strong hunger pangs by eating the kind of food she felt would be really satisfying – like bread spread with brie. After three weeks, she'd kept off the two kilos she'd lost before her weight loss stalled – and dropped another extra kilo.

'Before, I would have tried to work through the plateau by eating more vegetables to quash my hunger, and moving more, but I found that the key was to eat satisfying wholesome food instead,' she says. 'If I was really hungry and felt like lasagne, that's what I ate.'

Sainsbury-Salis had uncovered what she calls the famine reaction, a survival mechanism that can kick in when the body recognises that it's taking in fewer kilojoules.

'Your body slows down your metabolism, compensating for your lower kilojoule intake and priming you to store fat,' she explains.

To understand why, it helps to remember that humans didn't evolve in a landscape littered with food outlets, but in an environment with an uncertain food supply – that's why the body can't distinguish between a weight loss diet and a famine. This explains why, like many others, Sainsbury-Salis found that with every attempt at weight loss, she'd gain weight as her metabolism slowed down.

Still, not everyone who tries to lose weight will have a famine reaction, she says.

'Genes play a role. There are some people who have a strong famine reaction – and some who never have it, nor struggle with plateaus.'

Although Sainsbury-Salis' message is to not restrict food, it's no licence to pig-out either. Her advice is to follow a sensible weight loss plan based on mainly wholefoods and being physically active – but to also recognise genuine hunger and feed it with real food. This lets the body know the 'famine' is over and restores brain chemistry to normal. Like me, she also emphasises eating a wide variety of unprocessed foods.

'Research shows that not getting enough nutrients because you're eating less can rev up your appetite and make you want to eat more – a way of forcing you to find missing nutrients,' she says. 'Most foods you eat should be as close as possible to their natural state. Some studies in rats show that long-term consumption of foods high in fat and sugar can also provoke a famine reaction, possibly because the body recognises it's not getting the nutrients it needs.'

Have a healthier relationship with food

If food is hard to resist and you have difficulty shedding weight, think about what makes you eat. Is it raw, hollow stomach hunger or because you're sad, angry, stressed or even bored?

For some people, stress acts like an appetite killer, and for others it drives them to eat more – and it's often foods like muffins or Mars Bars. Although there's some willpower involved here, there may be biological factors that weaken our resolve. One theory suggests that stress chemicals raise levels of a brain chemical that stimulates eating, called neuropeptide Y (or NPY), and that NPY triggers a particular urge for carbohydrates. Or it may be that sweet foods cue our brains to produce feel-good chemicals like natural opiates or dopamine.

If you think you eat in response to stress or emotions, a food diary logging what you eat and what happened before you ate it will help you recognise the triggers. Or at least try and be aware of what's happening to make you eat. If it's anger, a low mood or stress, go for a walk if you can – even around the block will do (exercise can be a mood lifter and a stressbuster). If you're eating to numb a feeling, then, again, try a walk, or do some stretches, or take some deep breaths and make a cup of tea. Strategies like these can help you train yourself to find non-food ways to deal with feelings.

When you're fighting to resist overeating, or eating food you don't need, self-talk can sometimes help. Ask yourself what you would like most – the food in your mouth, or to off-load the roll of fat around your waist?

Taming night-time snacking

Too much grazing at night can set you up for a cycle of snacking that's hard to break. Snacking late at night can make you feel less like eating breakfast the next day – and more likely to snack later. It's better to try to eat more during the day so you're less likely to graze at night. If snacking in front of TV has become a habit, then watch less – or find something else to do while you watch (like knitting). If it's boredom snacking, find something that keeps you occupied – do a yoga class, learn something new, walk the dog or phone a friend.

What about treats?

Aim for quality rather than quantity. Have one fabulous chocolate or a small serving of your favourite cake occasionally and really enjoy it. More importantly, if you do break out and eat too much of the wrong thing, don't waste time on a guilt trip – go for a walk instead.

You only live once – so how about living smarter?

You know those people who justify their chips-with-everything approach with the phrase, you only live once? 'You only live once, so bring on the bacon.' 'You only live once, so let's have another drink.'

But the point is, we *do* only live once, so wouldn't it make sense to be smart about it? More than one in every three cancer deaths worldwide, for instance, is caused by nine risk factors we can do something about – including being overweight, low fruit and vegetable intake, physical inactivity and alcohol – say researchers from the Harvard School of Public Health. A cleaner lifestyle doesn't come with a guarantee of evading killer diseases but they can improve your odds. You can't control your genes but you can control what you eat and how active you are. So why not eat and exercise for your life – and your waistline too?

How will you look and move in decades to come?

A really striking woman is sitting two chairs away from me at the hairdresser and even though she's well into her 70s, she's a head-turner – thick, beautiful hair, flattering make-up and expensive, well-cut clothes. She looks wonderful, until she starts to move slowly and hesitantly towards the door and you realise how frail she is under her designer jacket, and how stiff her movements are.

As a race, we are living longer, and what you do with your body now can have a big impact on not just how you look, but on how well you'll function in your 70s, 80s and 90s. Stare into the future for a minute and imagine yourself at 75 or 85. Will you struggle to stand up because you've lost strength in the muscles that help propel you out of a chair? Will you be reaching for a Zimmer frame, or will you still be bushwalking and carrying your own shopping? Even without a crystal ball, there's every chance that, unless you commit to regular exercise between now and then, much of your body's muscle will have been replaced by fat, and your bones will be thinner. Not only will this affect how you look – droopier – but how efficiently your body works.

Let's think about this for a minute because it's important. With weaker muscles, and they *will* get weaker if you do nothing, how easily will you be able to do all the things that you take for granted now, like bending, balancing, squatting to pick something up off the floor, lifting a heavy bag, stretching to reach a high shelf? Will you be able to climb the stairs? You may have never thought about this stuff – most people don't. This is where there's a yawning gap in our thinking about the future. We're trained to prepare for our financial security as we get older, but how many of us plan ahead for our functional security? Yet keeping to a healthy weight and being active can go a long way towards preventing – or at least delaying – the onset of physical disability as we age.

When the World Health Organization's first woman director-general, Gro Harlem Brundtland, was in office not long ago she summed up the health of the world very neatly: people in some parts of the world are living dangerously because they have no choice, she said – and some people are living dangerously because they make the wrong choices. The kind of choices we make about how we live, eat and spend our spare time have a lot to do with our health, and our looks, as we move into our 40s and older. What kind of choices are you going to make?

Where to get more help

Eating

* The *Dietitians Association of Australia* – www.daa.asn.au
* *SMART Recovery* A self help, non-profit program that helps people find practical ways to cope with addictive behaviours that involve food, alcohol and other drugs, as well as gambling. Their website, www.smartrecoveryaustralia.com.au, has information on meetings in Australia.
* *Overeaters Anonymous* has a 12-step program to help people cope with overeating. Their website, www.oa.org.au, has details of meetings in Australia.
* To find out the GI of different foods, go to the *Glycemic Index* website at www.glycemicindex.com.

Fitness

* *Fitness Australia* is the professional organisation of the fitness industry. See their website, www.fitnessaustralia.com.au, for details of an accredited gym, fitness centre or personal trainer in your area.
* *Australian Association for Exercise and Sports Science*. The professional organisation of exercise physiologists. An exercise physiologist can design an exercise program suitable for anyone with an injury or medical condition (e.g. diabetes, heart disease or arthritis). People diagnosed with a range of health problems including high cholesterol, diabetes, arthritis and depression can claim a Medicare rebate from consultations with an exercise physiologist. The AAESS website can help you locate a practitioner in your area – see www.aaess.com.au.

Mental wellbeing

* *The Australian Psychological Association* To find a psychologist in your area, go to the APS website at www.psychology.org.au.

Women's health at menopause

* *The Jean Hailes Foundation for Women's Health* is a good source of credible information on women's health, sexual health, nutrition and wellbeing at menopause. See their website at www.jeanhailes.org.au.

For more good reading

The *Strong Women* series by Dr Miriam Nelson, including *Strong Women Stay Young; Strong Women Stay Slim; Strong Women, Strong Bones; Strong Women, Strong Hearts* (Lothian)

The Body in Action – the 'bible' of stretching, by physiotherapist Sarah Keys (Allen & Unwin)

Acknowledgements

Journalists are only as good as their sources of information. I'm grateful for the input of the many experts who've contributed to my knowledge of fitness, nutrition and women's health, as well as the women who shared their fitness experiences with me, and I'd like to thank them all: Dr Rosemary Stanton, Dr Clare Collins, Dr Lauren Williams, Dr Wendy Brown, Susie Burrell, Sue Radd, Monica Kubizniak, Chris Tzar, Allan Bolton, Sally Hitchman, James Short, Heidi Dening, Corey Bocking, Tony Boutagy, Dr Maria Fiatarone Singh, Dr Miriam Nelson, Catherine Saxelby, Trent Watson, Dr Alan Barclay, Dr Jennie Brand-Miller, Dr Amanda Sainsbury-Salis, Dr Genevieve Healy, Dr Garry Egger, Dr Naomi Rogers, Delwyn Bartlett, Professor Flavia Cicuttini, Annie Crawford, Martha Lourey-Bird, Kate Marsh, Karen Miller-Kovach, Rhonda Anderson, Greer Shipley, Professor Helena Teede, Sandra Villella, Sheryl Macrow-Cain, Bev Hadgraft, Wendy Guest, Sally Turansky, Dr Jane Givney, Susan Nicholson, Anne Riches, Lee-Anne Carson, Sue Sutton and Elizabeth Adams.

I'd also like to thank *Fit & Firm*'s cover girl, Jenny O'Toole, who is living proof of how effective the right food and exercise can be at midlife.